A STEP-BY STEP MA

FIRST AID

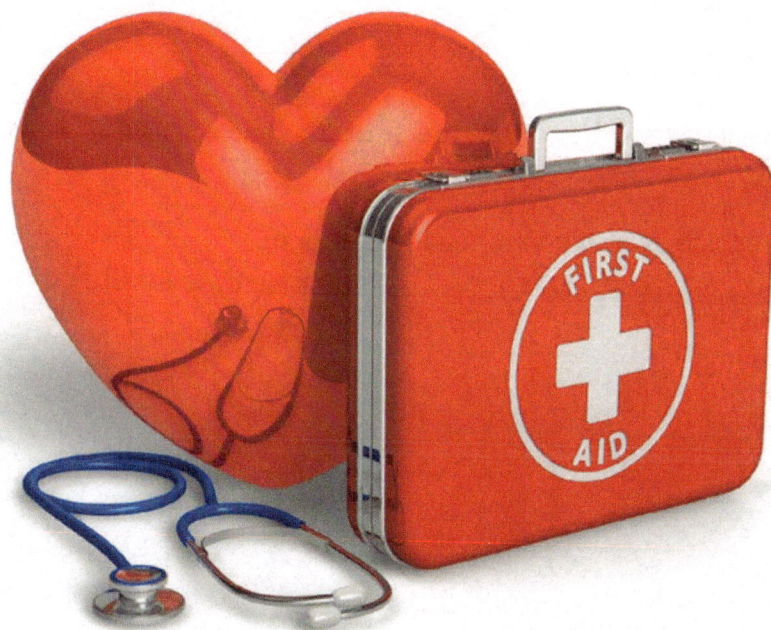

BLESSING ISAACKSON

DISCLAIMER

The author, Blessing Isaackson, and the publisher, Fairview Training Ltd, have made every effort to ensure that the information, tables, drawings, and diagrams contained in this book are accurate at the time of publication. The book cannot always contain all the information necessary for determining appropriate care and cannot address all individual situations; therefore, anyone using this book must ensure they have the appropriate knowledge and skills to enable suitable interpretation. The author does not guarantee and accepts no legal liability of whatever nature arising from or connected to, the accuracy, reliability, currency, or completeness of the content in this book. Users must always be aware that innovations or alterations after the date of publication may not be incorporated into the content. The author and the publisher assume no responsibility for the content of external resources in the text or accompanying online materials.

Printing History First Edition 2024

The author welcomes feedback from the users of this book. Please email your feedback to bisaackson@gmail.com

The CIP record for this book is available from the British Library.

Paperback ISBN: 978-1-7385061-4-9

eBook ISBN: 978-1-7385061-4-9

FOREWORD

The author, Blessing Isaackson, is the Managing Director of Fairview Training Ltd, the parent company of First Aid Tutors. He is an experienced trainer, assessor, and quality assurer. He is also the author of the following books: Immediate Life Support for Healthcare Practitioners – A Step-by-Step Guide, Managing Medical Emergencies in a Dental Practice, Immediate Life Support for Dental Workers – A Step-by-Step Guide, Education and Training Manual, Basic Life Support for Healthcare Practitioners, Basic Life Support for Dental workers, First Aid – A Step-by-Step Manual, and Fire Safety for Vehicle Drivers.

Fairview Training is committed to providing excellent resources for our learners, aiming to assist them in achieving their qualifications.

This book has been written to help learners to provide First Aid in all environments.

Learners can use this material during the training and as a reference even when they have completed the course.

Blessing Isaackson

Managing Director

Fairview Training Ltd

CONTENTS

FIRST AID

First aid are the actions that you take to help someone before the emergency services arrive.

Aims of first aid

The aims of a first aider are:

P – Preserve the casualty's life.
P – Prevent the casualty's condition from getting worse.
P – Promote the recovery of the casualty.

YOUR ROLE AS A FIRST AIDER

ASSESS THE ENVIRONMENT

Make sure you are safe and the casualty is not exposed to any further harm.

PRIORITISE TREATMENT

Where there are multiple injuries involving multiple casualties, always treat the most serious injuries first. If any of the casualties are not breathing, treat them first and then approach any bleeding casualties. Catastrophic bleeding should always be treated urgently, otherwise, there is a risk that they might bleed to death.

GET HELP

If you are on your own and you have access to a phone, call 999/112 for assistance. If there is a bystander with you, they should call the emergency services.

WHAT YOU SHOULD TELL THE OPERATOR

• Give the operator your number.

• Tell them where you are and the condition of the casualty.

SEEK THE CONSENT OF THE CASUALTY

Ask for permission from the casualty before treating him/her. Consent is implied if the casualty is unconscious.

MINIMISE THE RISK OF INFECTION

• Wear gloves.

• Wash your hands and place a face shield on the casualty's face when performing CPR.

• Wear Personal Protective Equipment (PPE).

• Hand hygiene.

- Dispose of contaminated waste.

- Use appropriate dressings.

- Wear barrier devices during rescue breaths.

 - Cover any of your own cuts

QUALITIES OF AN EFFECTIVE FIRST AIDER

- Calmness.
- Vigilance – be aware of the risks around you. Make sure you and the casualty are safe.
- Build and maintain trust between you and the casualty.
- Stick to your limitations. Do not exceed your limits.
- If you have not been trained to conduct a treatment, do not experiment.

SCENE SURVEY

Make sure you check the scene for anything that may cause harm to you or the patient or any bystander. Look around the patient for broken glass, bodily fluid, exposed electrical wiring, gas, fire, and traffic.

You should:
- Ensure it is safe to provide help to the patient.
- Find out what happened.
- Count the number of casualties.
- Assess whether the EMS will be required.
- Ensure you have the required PPE (Personal Protective Equipment).
- Check if you have an AED.

Assess the patient.
Only provide help when it is safe to do so.
While assessing the patient, introduce yourself, and if they fail to respond, call 999/112.

An Unconscious and Non-Breathing Patient

If you are alone and the patient is unconscious and not breathing, then call for help immediately, then start CPR.

If you are with the patient and have other helpers around, send one of the helpers to call 999/112 and to also bring an AED.

ILLNESS ASSESSMENT

To effectively assess an ill patient, it is important to follow the mnemonic S.A.M.P.L.E:

S – Signs and Symptoms: Temperature, skin colour, pulse rate. Only the patient can tell you their symptoms, so ask them questions to find out.

A – Allergies: Is the patient allergic to anything?

M – Medication: Is the patient taking any medication?

P – Past Medical History: Does the patient have any medical conditions?

L – Last Meal/Fluid: When did the patient last eat or drink?

E – Event History: What was the event leading up to the patient becoming ill?

PRIMARY SURVEY

D – Danger
R – Response
A – Airway
B – Breathing
C – Circulation

AIRWAY

Make sure the casualty's airway is clear and unobstructed. A casualty who is unresponsive cannot discharge vomit obstructing his airway, whereas a conscious casualty can. So, make sure an unconscious casualty has a clear airway. You can check their airway by tilting their head back and looking inside the casualty's mouth.

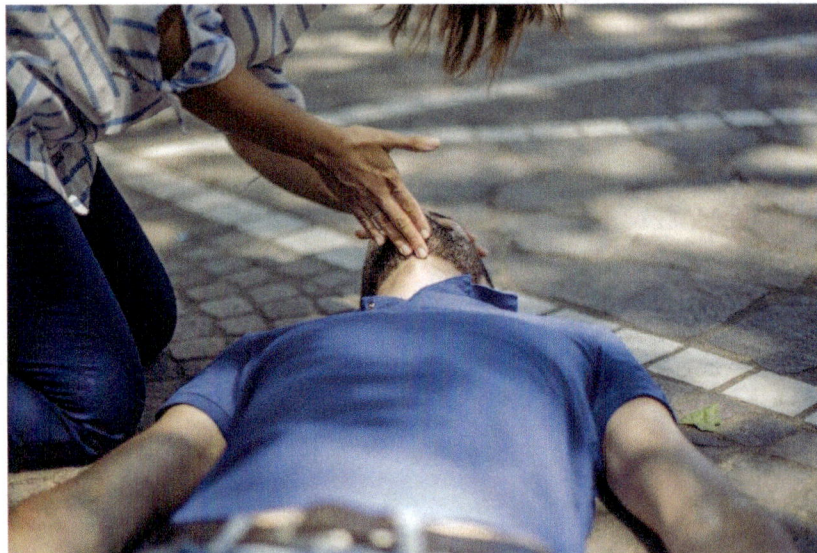

BREATHING

The primary survey involves checking if the casualty is breathing normally for about 10 seconds.

Look – Look at the chest and see if it is moving up and down.

Listen – Bring your cheek close to the cheek and listen for sounds of breathing.

Feel – Feel the breath on your cheek.

See – See the chest rise and fall.

 If the casualty is not breathing, call 999/112 immediately for emergency help. The next step is to look for any evidence of severe bleeding, but skip this step if the casualty is not breathing and you can clearly see he is not bleeding severely.

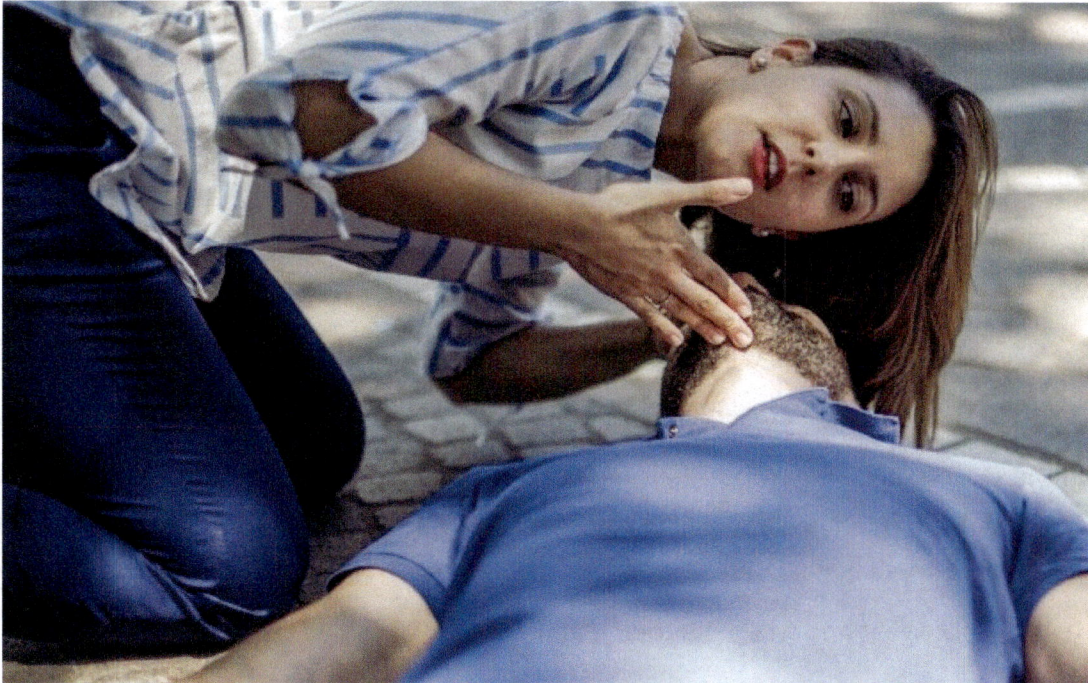

CIRCULATION

If the casualty is breathing normally, then you may proceed to the next stage, which is checking for evidence of severe bleeding. If the casualty is bleeding, this will require your immediate attention, otherwise, the casualty will suffer from shock—a condition that results in a breakdown of the circulatory system. Call 999/112 immediately if you suspect severe bleeding. In the absence of severe bleeding, you must conduct the secondary survey, which involves a more detailed form of assessment of the casualty.

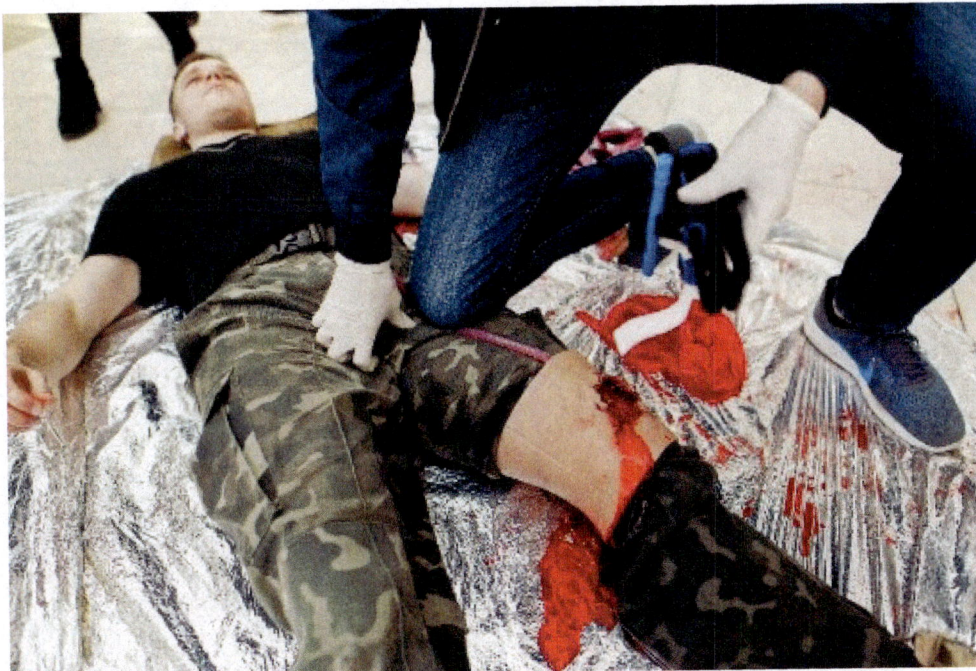

SECONDARY SURVEY

This occurs when you examine the casualty to find out other injuries or conditions that you may have either missed or did not notice when conducting the primary survey.

S – SIGNS: Injuries or any deformity that are apparent, e.g. sweating, vomit, anxiety, hot or cold skin, wheezing, alcohol, and urine.

SYMPTOMS: These are things that only the casualty can tell you about. E.g. pain, faintness, headache, and dizziness.

A – AIRWAY: Can the casualty tell you any allergies that they might have?

M – MEDICATION: Has the person taken any medications? If so, when?

P – PAST MEDICAL HISTORY: Finding out their medical history will give us an idea of the cause of the present illness. Look out for clues of the illness such as bracelets and necklaces, which will contain written clues of a pre-existing illness.

L – LAST MEAL/FLUID: What and when did the casualty last eat?

E – EVENT HISTORY: What happened?

SECONDARY SURVEY

Head to toe search

CLUES

MEDICAL BRACELETS

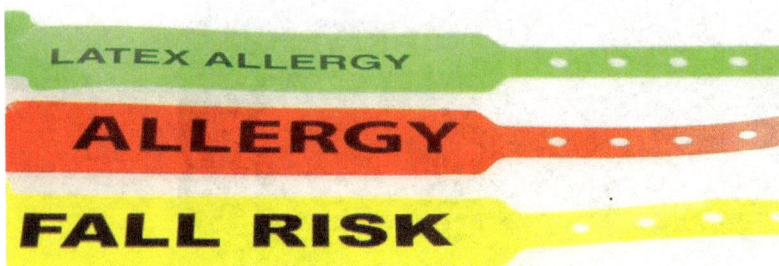

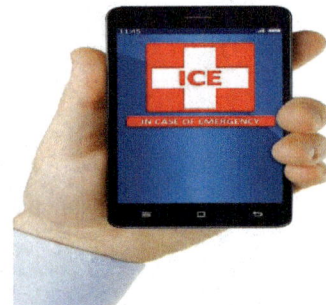

THE CHAIN OF SURVIVAL

This chain represents the steps that can be taken by the first aider to enhance the chances of a casualty who has suffered from a cardiac arrest.

STEP 1

EARLY RECOGNITION AND EARLY CALL FOR HELP

The common cause of a cardiac arrest in an adult is a heart attack. It is important to recognise the early signs, and one of the signs is a vice-like chest pain in the centre of the chest. If you can recognise a heart attack and treat it before the emergency services arrive, then you can stop a cardiac arrest. An early call for help is vital to the casualty's survival.

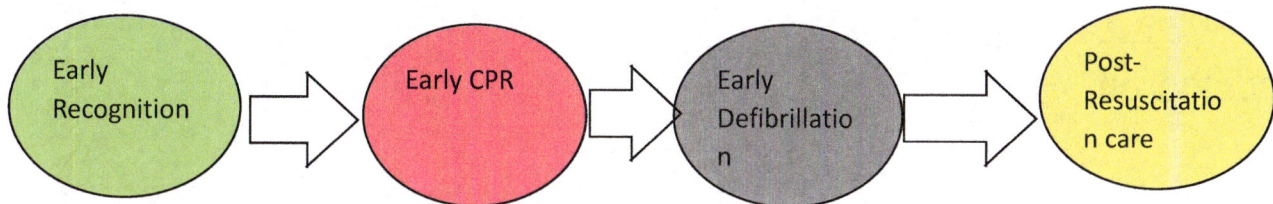

Early Recognition → Early CPR → Early Defibrillation → Post-Resuscitation care

STEP 2

EARLY CPR

CPR must commence as soon as you know the casualty is not breathing. This can, at the very least, double the chances of survival of the casualty. For every minute you wait, the chances of the casualty surviving decreases by 10%

STEP 3

EARLY DEFIBRILLATION

According to the UK Resuscitation Council, using the defibrillator on a cardiac arrest casualty within 3-5 minutes increases their survival rate by 50%-70%.

https://www.resus.org.uk/resuscitation-guidelines/adult-basic-life-support-and-automated-external-defibrillation/#chain.

STEP 4

POST-RESUSCITATION CARE

If bystander efforts have failed in reviving the casualty, then advanced life support care provided by the emergency services through airway management and administration of drugs can assist the casualty's recovery.

ANGINA

Angina is chest pain caused by reduced blood flow to the heart muscles. Angina can be stable—usually triggered by stress or exercise. This tends to get better when you rest.

Unstable angina is more unpredictable and more serious. It may happen without any known triggers and can occur even whilst at rest.

Angina is usually triggered by the narrowing of the arteries that supply blood to the heart muscles, typically caused by deposits of cholesterol plaque. As a result of the narrowing of the arteries, there is reduced blood supply to the heart. Angina is an indication that the casualty is at risk of a heart attack or stroke. The risk of a heart attack can be minimized through a change in lifestyle.

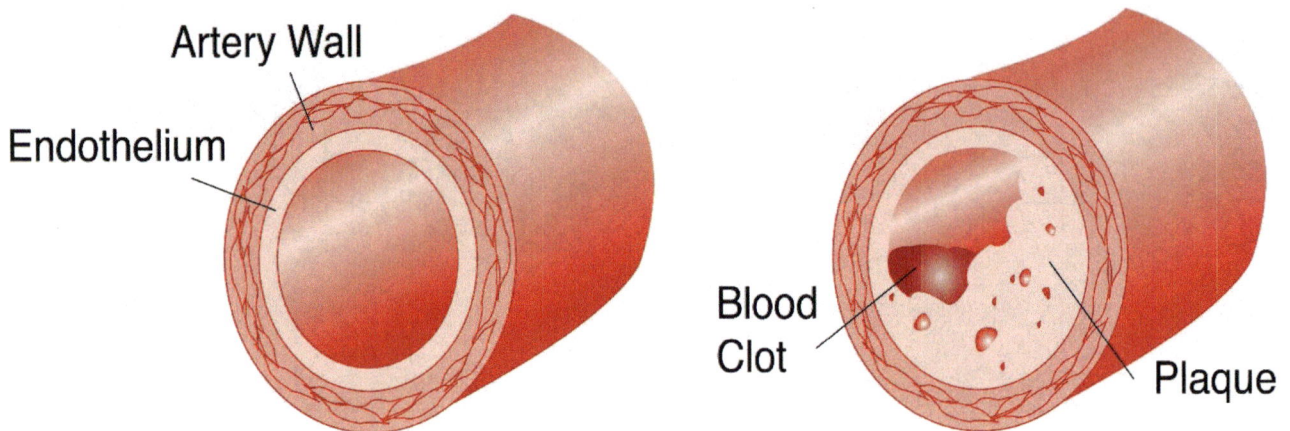

Normal Artery

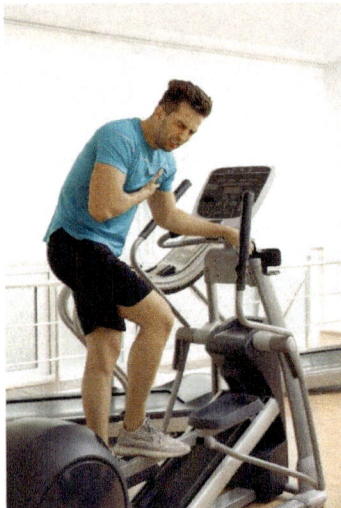

Diseased Artery

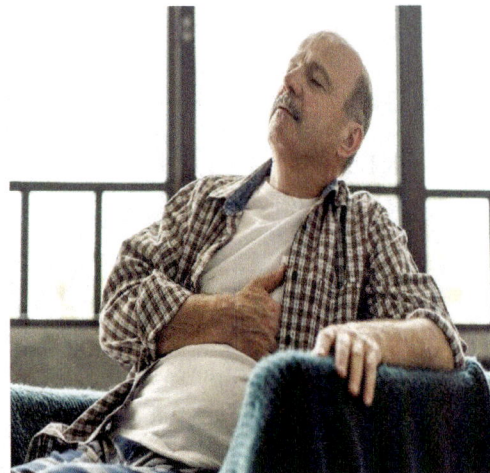

- Chest pain which will normally subside by resting and presents as tightness, dullness, or a heavy pain in the centre of the chest, which may

radiate to the arm—usually the left arm—neck, jaw, and back. The pain

should not last for more than 3-8 minutes. If it lasts longer, then suspect a heart attack.

Call 999/112 and get the AED ready.

Recognising Angina

- Chest pain triggered by physical exertion, change in the weather, and stress.
- Chest pain, which subsides by the patient resting.
- Pain in the centre of the chest, which radiates to the jaw, back, and shoulders.
- Nausea or vomiting.
- Breathlessness.
- Dizziness.
- Casualty is usually anxious.

TREATMENT OF ANGINA

• Get the casualty to rest in a comfortable position. Provide reassurance

to reduce anxiety and minimize the pain.

• Does the casualty take any medicines for the condition? If so, get them

to take it.

Administer GTN

Get the patient to rest in a comfortable position.

Provide reassurance to reduce anxiety and minimize the pain.

Ask the patient if he has a GTN spray or tablets with him and ask him to spray it under his tongue or take the tablets.

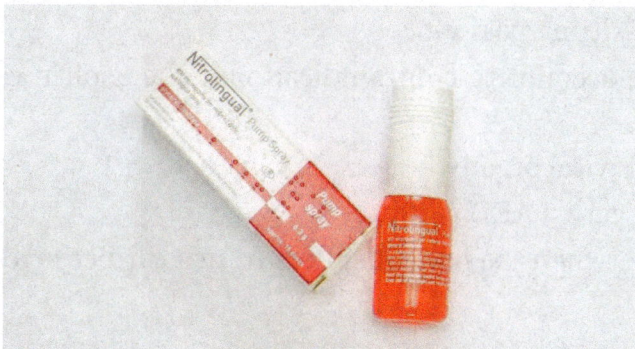

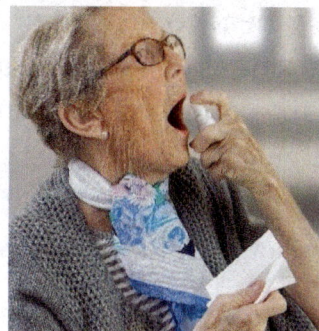

Heart Attack

Heart attack results from a blockage of the coronary arteries by cholesterol plaque. The breakage of the plaque leads to the development of a blood clot on the spot of breakage. The blood clot results in a sizeable number of cases to a complete blockage, which leads to sections supplied by the blocked coronary arteries dying. This may result in a heart attack.

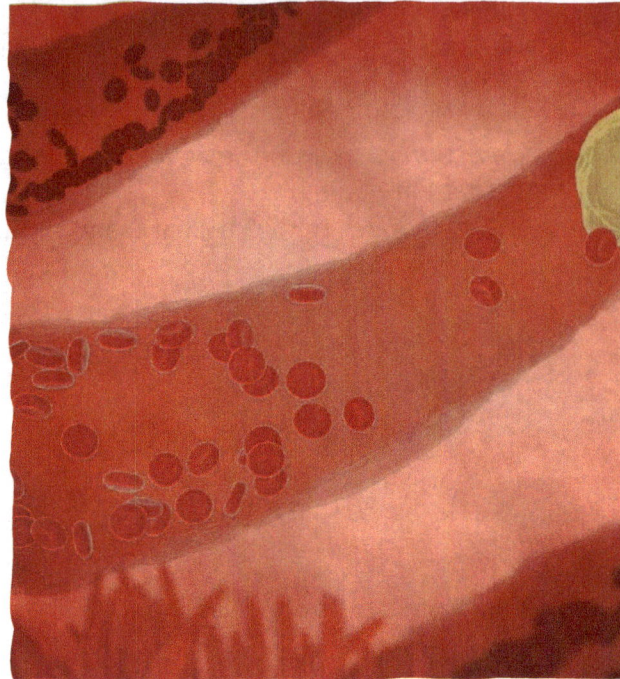

Signs and Symptoms of a Heart Attack

- A persistent vice-like and central chest pain, which does not ease with resting.
- Abdominal pain or a feeling of indigestion.
- Look out for a change in the colour of the casualty's skin. The casualty's skin might be pale or grey in colour. Their lips might be blue.
- Breathlessness and dizziness.
- Nausea and vomiting.
- A feeling of impending doom.

Treatment of a Heart Attack

- With early recognition of a heart attack, call 999/112.
- Calm the patient's anxiety.
- The patient needs to sit in a half-sitting position.
- Give 300mg of aspirin but take account of contraindications. The aspirin can be chewed or dissolved in water.
- Continue to monitor the patient's vital organs.
- Be ready to treat cardiac arrest—get an AED ready.
- Commence CPR and use the AED when the patient suffers from a cardiac arrest.

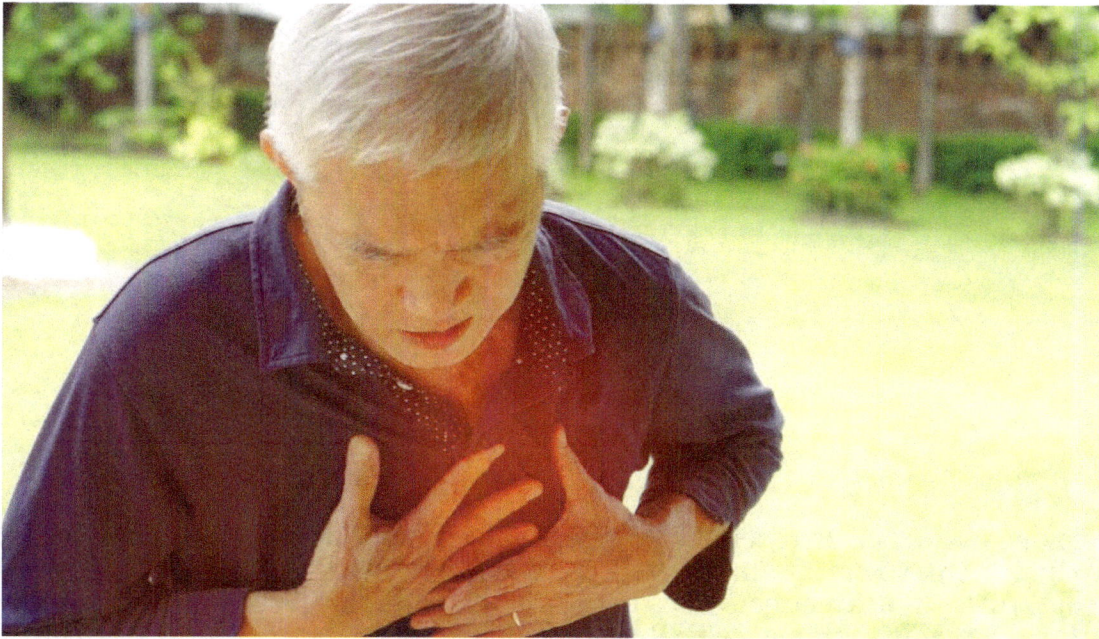

Choking

Choking occurs when there is a full or partial blockage of the airway. It occurs between the mouth and the carina—the part of the airway where the left and the right bronchi split from the bronchi.

Causes of Choking

- Eating too quickly.
- Extracted prosthesis.
- Eating whilst lying down.
- Not chewing food properly.
- Foreign objects.
- Teeth.
- Vomit.
- Root canal files.
- Dental burs.

Mild Choking

This happens when the airway is partly blocked. With partial blockage, the patient can still speak. In this case, you should encourage him to cough, and they should be able to clear the obstruction themselves. If the obstruction does clear, then commence the back blows.

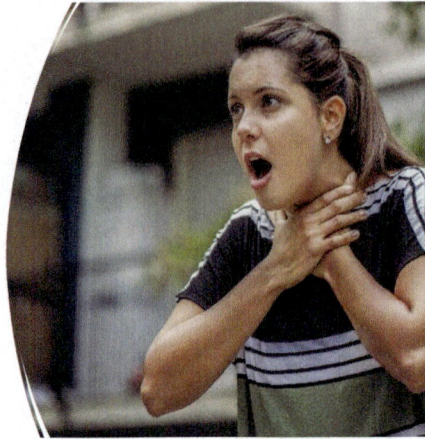

Severe Choking

Severe choking usually involves a full blockage of the airway. The person will not be able to speak. To help them, you must immediately commence five back blows followed by five abdominal thrusts. If the treatment does not work, the patient will become unconscious and not breathing. You must commence CPR immediately.

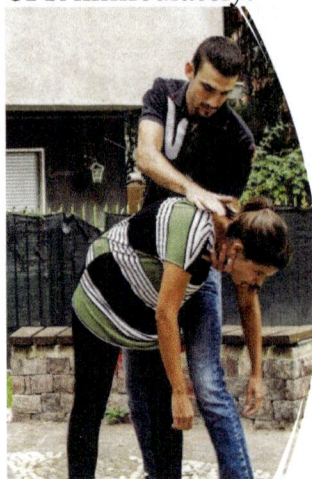

Abdominal Thrusts

Make a fist with your dominant hand and then place that fist above the navel and below the tip of the sternum. Press backwards and upwards up to five times.

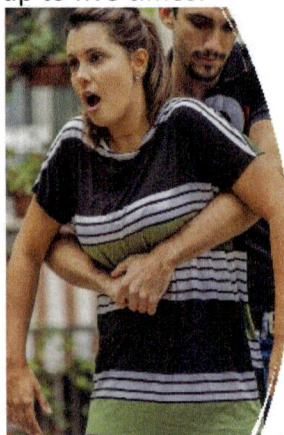

Choking Baby

Choking Infant – No Blind Finger Sweep

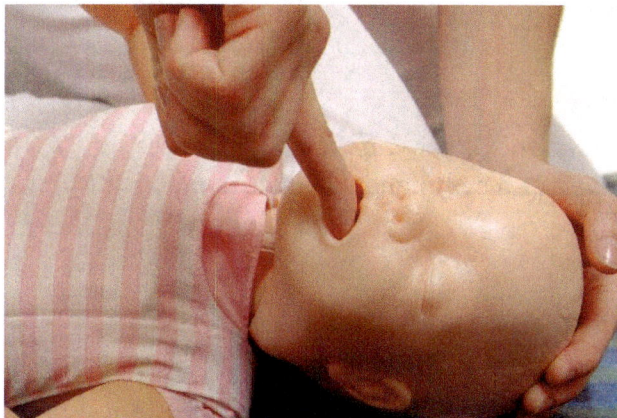

Choking Infant – Back Blows
Give up to 5 back blows using the heel of hand your dominant hand.

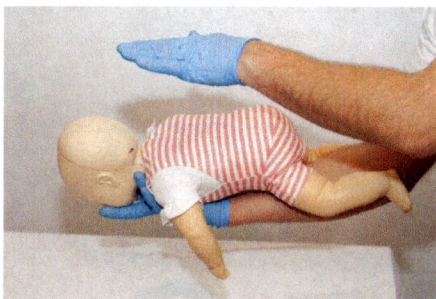

Choking Infant – Chest Thrust
After the 5 back blows, begin up to five chest thrusts with your index and middle fingers.

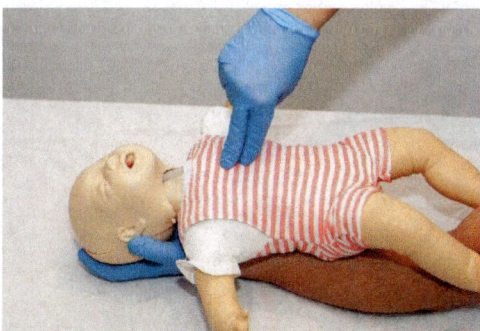

WHAT TO DO WHEN YOU FIND A COLLAPSED CASUALTY WHO IS RESPONSIVE

D – Danger: Check around for danger.

R – Response: Check for response—is the casualty alert? Can they hear your voice? Are they responding to pain? Shake the casualty's shoulder and give out a command – "Squeeze my hand!" "Open your eyes!"

IF THE CASUALTY RESPONDS-
Leave the casualty where you found them.

Check for any life-threatening injuries in order of priority.

Give priority to more serious injuries. If necessary, call for help and continue to monitor the casualty's vital signs until help arrives.

PRIORITY OF TREATMENT – Prioritise catastrophic bleeding over burns and burns over broken bones.

WHAT TO DO WHEN YOU FIND A COLLAPSED CASUALTY WHO IS UNRESPONSIVE

D – Danger: Check around for danger.

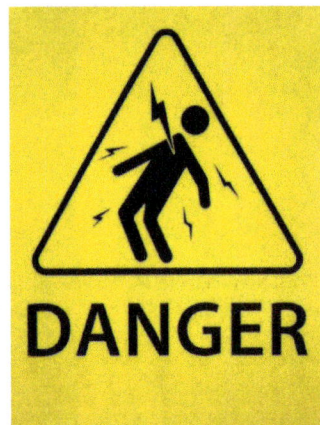

R – Response: Check for response—is the casualty alert? Can they hear your voice? Are they responding to pain? Shake the casualty's shoulder and give out a command – "Squeeze my hand!" "Open your eyes!"

IF THE CASUALTY IS UNRESPONSIVE

If the casualty is unresponsive, leave him where you found him and then:

S – Shout for help.

A – Airway: Check the airway—make sure the airway is clear by tilting it back.

B – Breathing: Check that the casualty has normal breathing—an average of 2-4 breaths in a minute.

C – Circulation: Check for signs of circulatory failure—heart attack, possible cardiac arrest, or bleeding.

TO REMEMBER THESE STEPS, REMEMBER DRS ABC.

BLEEDING

WHAT HAPPENS WHEN THERE IS AN INJURY?

The injured blood vessel narrows to reduce blood flow from the body.
The body produces a blood clot to stem the blood flow.

RULES OF DRESSING

WHAT YOU SHOULD NOT DO
Do not give someone with severe bleeding anything to eat or drink.

This is because it is safer to have an operation on an empty stomach. Someone with a severe bleed is likely to have an operation.

WHAT YOU SHOULD DO
Remove or cut away any clothing that might get in the way of dressing the wound.

Apply direct pressure to the wound with a sterile dressing or a clean, non-fluffy pad.

APPLYING DRESSING TO A BLEEDING ARM:

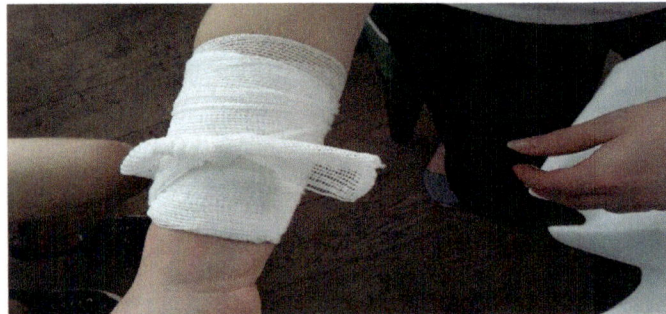

Do not wait for a dressing. Where there is no dressing, ask the casualty to apply pressure themselves, or you can help by applying direct pressure with your hands using a sterile non-fluffy pad.

WHERE THERE IS AN EMBEDDED OBJECT IN THE WOUND
Apply pressure on either side of the wound.

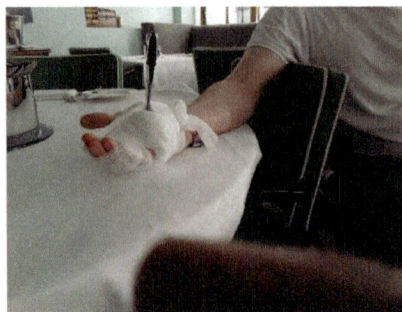

- Call 999/112 for emergency help.

- Secure the dressing with a bandage that will put pressure on the wound, but make sure the bandage is not too tight that it interferes with circulation.

- If the first dressing is soaked with blood, apply a second. If the second dressing is also soaked in blood, remove both dressings and apply a fresh one.

- Laceration: A deep cut to the skin or flesh. The bleeding in this type of wound is not as much as in an incised wound, but the damage is likely to be more severe. The likelihood of an infection is high because they are more susceptible to germs.

TYPES OF BLEEDING

- Arterial bleeding.
- Venous bleeding.
- Capillary bleeding.

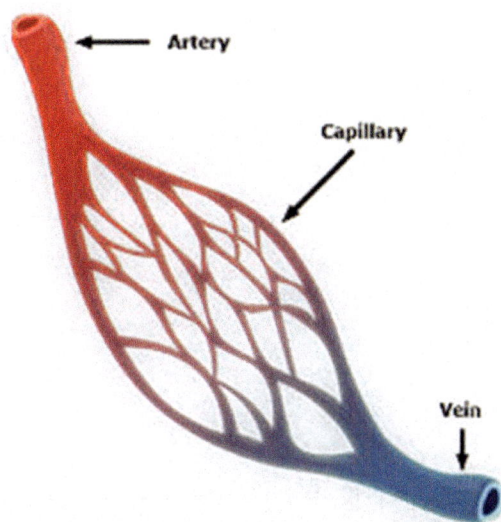

Arterial bleeding
The arteries transport oxygenated blood from the heart, and when the artery is damaged, blood spurts out of the wound every time the heart beats. The blood loss is very rapid, and life could be threatened within a matter of two minutes because the volume of blood falls quite rapidly. The colour of the blood is bright red.

Venous bleeding
Carries deoxygenated blood to the heart, and because it has given up the oxygen in the blood to the body tissues, the colour of the blood is darker red. It is not under the same amount of pressure that you will find in the arteries, but the volume of blood remains the same, and bleeding can, therefore, be profuse.

Capillary bleeding

Bleeding from the capillaries occurs in every wound and it would initially be quite profuse, but the blood loss is slight and can be controlled quite easily.

What blood loss is normal, and what effects does it have on the body?

Loss of 10% blood volume/0.5 litres (about one pint):
- The level of consciousness will be normal.
- The colour of the skin will be normal.
- The pulse will be normal.
- Breathing will be normal.
- This level of blood loss has no effect on the body.

Dangerous blood loss

Loss of 20% blood volume:

- May experience dizziness if they stand.
- Skin might become pale.
- The pulse will be slightly raised as would the breathing.

Loss of about three ½ pints of blood:

- Pulse quickens.
- Sweating.
- Shock develops.

Loss of 30% blood volume:
- Impaired consciousness.
- Restlessness.
- Anxiety.
- Grey-blue tinge to the lips, skin, earlobes, and nail beds.
- Rapid pulse.
- Rapid breathing.

Loss of 40% blood volume:
- The casualty will become unresponsive.
- Skin will be grey-blue, cold, and clammy.
- Pulse will be undetectable.
- Breathing will be deep.

CONTROLLING CATASTROPHIC BLEEDING

Ask the patient to apply direct pressure to the wound.

Call 999/112.

Apply a gauze pad or pressure dressing to the point of injury.

If the first dressing is ineffective in stopping the flow of blood, apply a second dressing.

Elevate the injured limb with an elevated sling.

HAEMOSTATIC DRESSINGS
Use haemostatic dressing to speed the clotting in the severe bleeding.

Do not use haemostatic dressings on an open head wound or open chest wounds. They are best for abdominal wounds or those in junctional parts of the body, such as the groin and armpit.

TOURNIQUET

Use a tourniquet if you are trained to use one to stop blood flow from the point of injury.

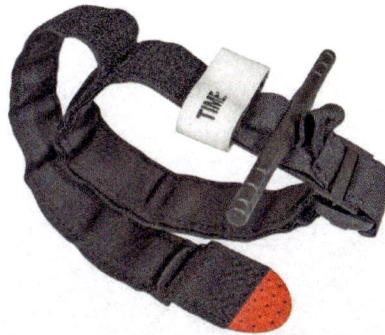

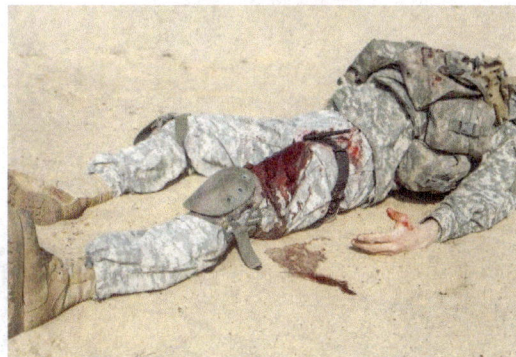

MINOR INJURIES

Flail chest injury.
This happens when portions of the rib cage is separated from other parts of the chest. The ribs are broken in several places due to severe blunt force or trauma. The affected ribs are not able to contribute to the expansion of the lungs which unfortunately means that the patient's breathing is affected.

Mechanics of a Flail Chest
When a patient with flail chest breaths in the abdomen rather than expand out is drawn in and when he breaths out the abdomen drawn in rather than out. This is referred to paradoxical breathing.

Symptoms
Paradoxical movement
Bruises
Grazes
Discolouration in the chest area

First Aid for Flail Chest Injury
Get the patient to seat upright and lean them towards the injured side.
Place a pillow or similar object under the patient arm.

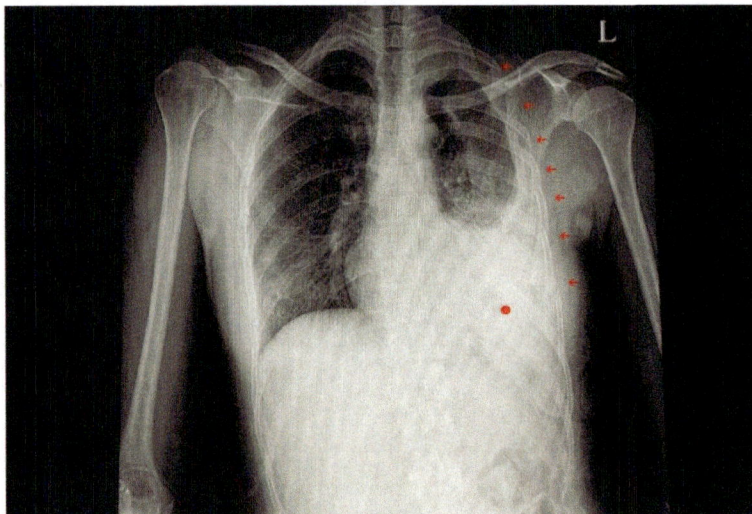

Knocked Out Adult Tooth

If a tooth is knocked out, replant it in the socket immediately and then get the patient to press down on a pad between the upper and bottom teeth to ensure the tooth is in place. Alternatively, ask the patient to keep it inside their cheek.

Apply a cold compress to the outside of the mouth to reduce any swelling.

You may put the tooth in a container of milk to stop it from becoming dry.

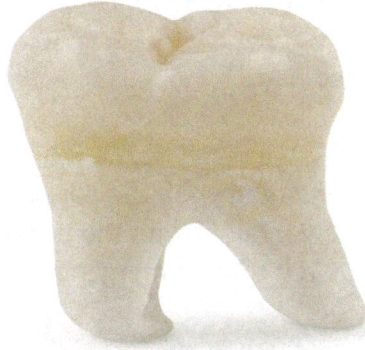

Evisceration (Disembowelment)

- Removal of internal organs, especially those in the abdominal cavity.
- Treatment.
- Call 999/112.
- Cover the wound with a clean, moist dressing.
- Do not attempt to push organs or bowels back in place.
- Monitor the patient for shock.

BRUISING

This occurs when there is bleeding beneath the tissues of the skin. It can appear days after an injury. Elderly patients and those who are on anti-coagulants are prone to bruising easily.

Raise and support the patient's injured part in a comfortable position and place cold compress on the injured area.

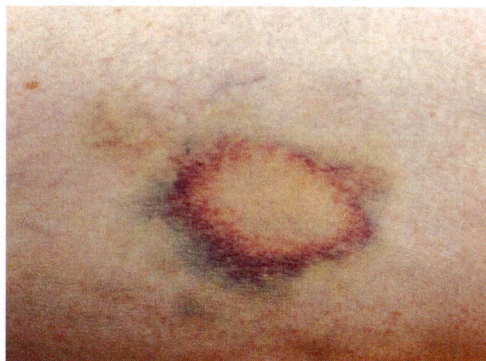

AMPUTATION

A limb that has been partially or fully detached from the body can be reattached through surgery if the patient can get to the hospital on time.

FIRST AID

Do not give food or drink to the patient.

Stop the flow of blood by applying direct pressure on the part injured and raise the injured part above the heart.

Apply a non-fluffy dressing on the inured part.

Call 999/112

Wrap the detached limb in a cling film and then wrap the package in a piece of gauze and then place in a container of crushed ice. It helps if the container with the package lim is labelled with the patient's name and the time of the injury and hand it to the Emergency medical service when they arrive.

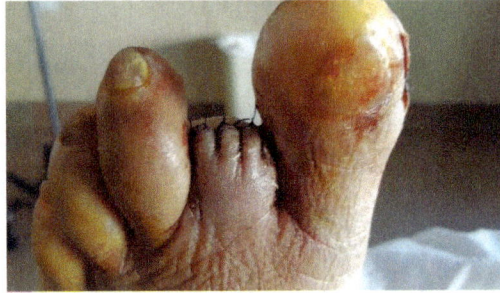

LACERATION

Laceration is a deep cut or tear in the skin. They can be caused by sharp objects such as scissors and knives.

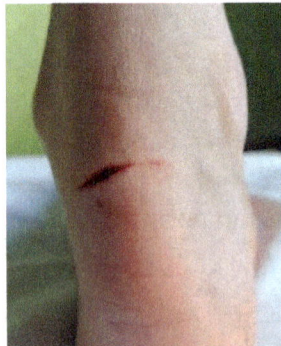

NOSEBLEED

CAUSES

Rupturing of tiny blood vessels in the nostrils due to physical trauma, picking the nose, blowing the nose, anti-blood clotting medicines.

FIRST AID

STEP 1

Ask patient to sit down with head tilted forward and pinch the soft part of their nose whilst breathing through the mouth. This should be done for about 10 minutes.

STEP 2
The patient should avoid coughing, talking, spitting or sniffing to prevent the dislodgment of blood clot that has already formed behind the squeezed nostrils.

STEP 3
If the patient's nostrils are still bleeding after the first 10 minutes, ask them to repeat the treatment by applying pressure on the nostrils for an additional 10 minutes. If this does not help, a further squeezing of the nose for a further 10 minutes will be required.

STEP 4
If the bleeding does not stop after 30 minutes then then the arrange to take or send the the patient to the hospital.

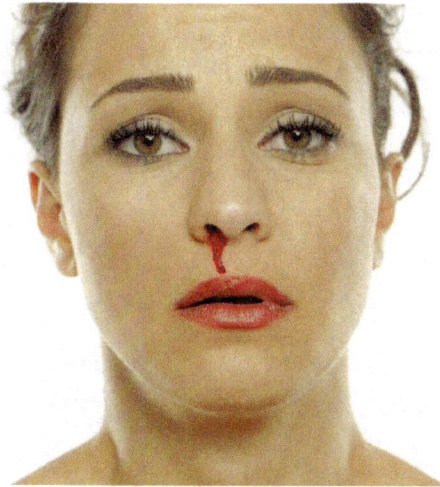

GRAZE

Step 1
Wash your hands and make sure they are dry and if you have gloves then wear them to minimise the risk of infection.

Step 2
Irrigate the wound with water or with sterile wipes to remove any dirt.

Step 3
Pat the wound and the area around the wound dry with a clean tea towel

Step 4
Put on a sterile dressing or plaster.

CRUSH INJURY

Crush injuries normally occur because of traffic or construction site accidents. The injuries may involve bleeding, fracture, and less visible internal injuries. If the patient is crushed for a prolonged period this may lead to severe damage to body tissues.

Prolonged crushing can also lead to "crush syndrome"- where toxins built up around the muscles because of the crushing is released suddenly into the circulatory system causing kidney failure or cardiac arrest.

LESS THAN 15 MINUTES
If you can confirm that the patient has been crushed for less than 15 minutes and it is safe to do so, then release them quickly, control any bleeding and stabilise the suspected fractured limb.

OVER 15 MINUTES
I the patient has been crushed for over 15 minutes and you or you cannot move object that led to the crushing then leave them where you found them. Provide comfort and reassure them. Immediately call 999/112. Provide them with as much details as possible. Continue to monitor the vital signs of the patient until the Emergency Medical Services arrive.

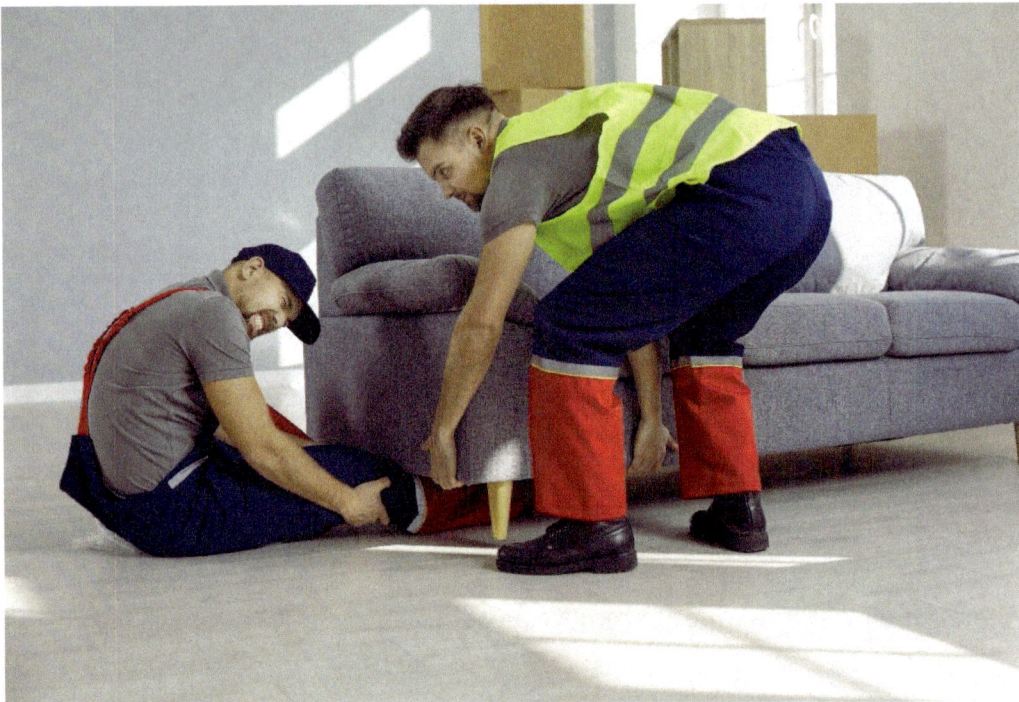

SPLINTER

What to do to help someone with a splinter in their finger.

Splinters can be made of wood, metal, or glass and can be quite painful when they penetrate the skin. Apart from the pain they cause, they carry the risk of infection to the affected area.

TREATMENT OF SPLINTERS

- Wash the finger with warm soapy water.

- Hold the splinter with tweezers close to the end and close to the skin.

- Pull the splinter out from the direction that it went into the skin. Be careful to avoid breakage.

- Once the splinter has been removed, squeeze the affected area to encourage bleeding to ensure any dirt in the wound is flushed out.

- Clean and dry the wound with a sterile dressing.

- Do not dislodge any splinter lodged in the skin with sharp objects.

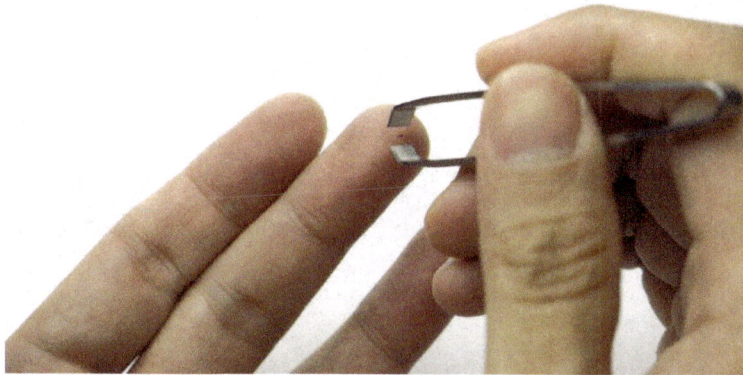

SMALL CUTS

Step 1
Wash your hands and make sure they are dry and if you have gloves then wear them to minimise the risk of infection.

Step 2
Irrigate the wound with water or with sterile wipes.

Step 3
Pat the wound and the area around the wound dry with a clean tea towel

Step 4
Put on a sterile dressing or plaster.

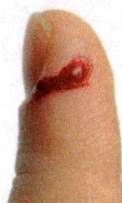

PENETRATING CHEST WOUND

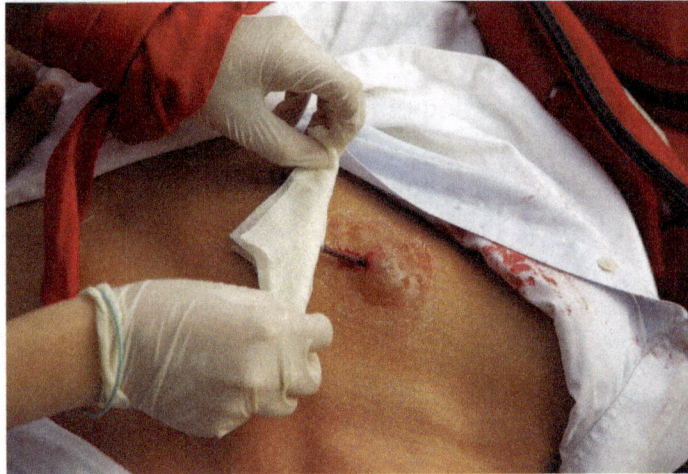

CAUSES
Sharp objects in the penetrative chest wall.

CONSEQUENCES

Damage to the lungs.

Damage to the pleura (the two-layered membrane that surrounds and protects the lungs).

PNEUMOTHORAX

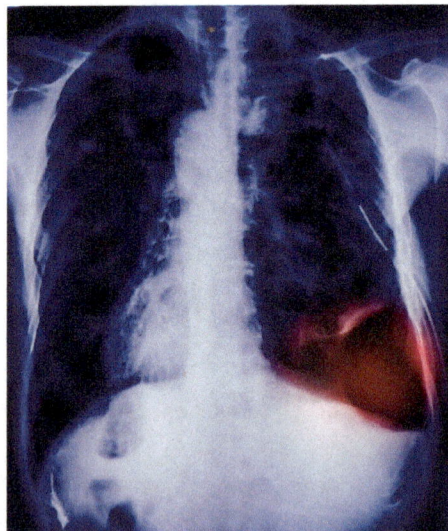

When the membranes are perforated, air enters and is trapped between the membranes and creates pressure on the lungs, which may collapse as a result. This condition is referred to as pneumothorax.

TENSION PNEUMORTHORAX

Pressure in the damaged lungs affects the uninjured lungs leading to difficulty breathing and this, in addition, may prevent the heart from refilling with blood. This affects the circulatory system and shock could be a consequence. This condition is called tension pneumothorax.

BLEEDING CHEST WOUND

Add direct pressure and cover the wound with a non-adhesive dressing.

NON-BLEEDING CHEST WOUND

Leave the wound exposed to the element without dressing.

WHAT TO DO

Sit the casualty down and support and lean them to the side of the injury.
If the wound is bleeding, control it with direct pressure and apply dressing if necessary.

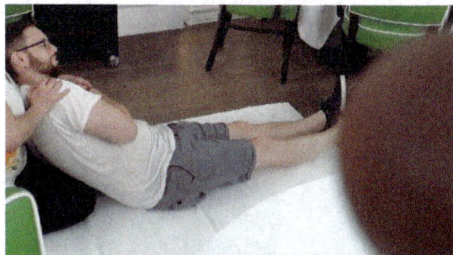

Call 999/112

Monitor and record vital signs.

If unresponsive but breathing, roll casualty on the injured side so the working of the good lung is not compromised.

RECOGNITION

- Rapid, shallow, and uneven breathing.
- Nervousness/a sense of doom.
- Hypoxia/Cyanosis.
- Coughing of frothy red blood.
- Crackling sound around the area of the wound.
- Blood bubbling out of the wound.
- Suckling sound as casualty breathes in air.
- Veins in the neck become prominent.

BURNS

CAUSES OF BURN

CHEMICAL BURN

Chemicals that can cause burns are:
Acid, paint stripper, caustic soda; weed killers; bleach; oven cleaner, and industrial chemicals.

ICE BURN

Frostbite
Any contact with freezing materials and contact with freezing vapours, for example, liquid oxygen and liquid nitrogen.

DRY BURN

Examples of a dry burn:
Flames, cigarettes, and friction (this can be caused by crawling on a carpet with the knees).

ELECTRICAL BURN

Examples:
Low voltage current.
High voltage current.
Lightning strikes.

RADIATION BURN

Sunburn
Ultraviolet rays from a sun lamp—exposure to an X-ray.

DEPTH OF BURNS

The depth of burns can be classified into:

SUPERFICIAL THICKNESS BURN- this is when the top layer of the skin is affected by the burn. They are painful, red and dry.

PARTIAL THICKNESS-damage to to the uppermost layer of the skin. These burns have blisters and are painful.

FULL THICKNESS—this involves damage to all the layers of the skin including the subcutaneous tissues.

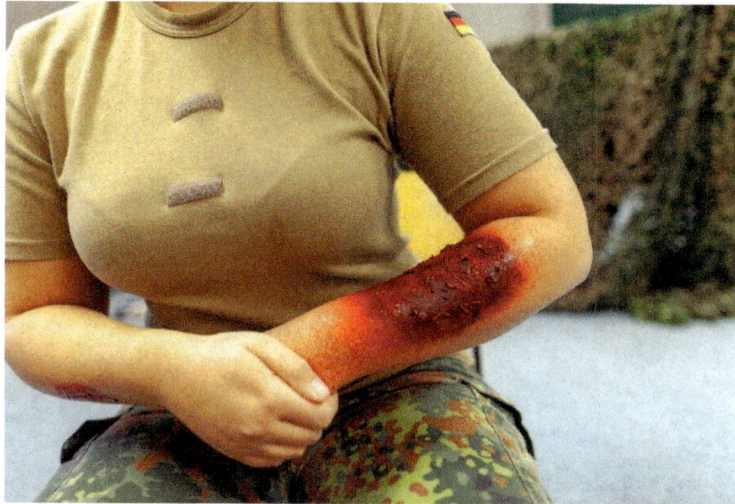

TREATMENT OF BURNS

Cool the burn with running water for 20 minutes. Remove any pieces of clothing or jewelry around the area of the burn. Do not use ice or iced water.
Cover the burn with a piece of cling film. If it is around the arm, you may use a clean plastic bag.

If the eyes or airway are affected get the patient to sit upright and not lying down.

WHEN TO GET THE PATIENT TO THE HOSPITAL

Whenever the burn has been caused by chemicals or electricity.

Large deep burns

Full thickness burns

When children and elderly patients have suffered burns.

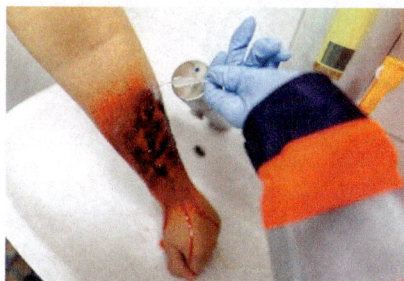

USE CLING FILM
Use cling film to wrap the burnt part of the body but do this loosely. Do not wrap too tightly.

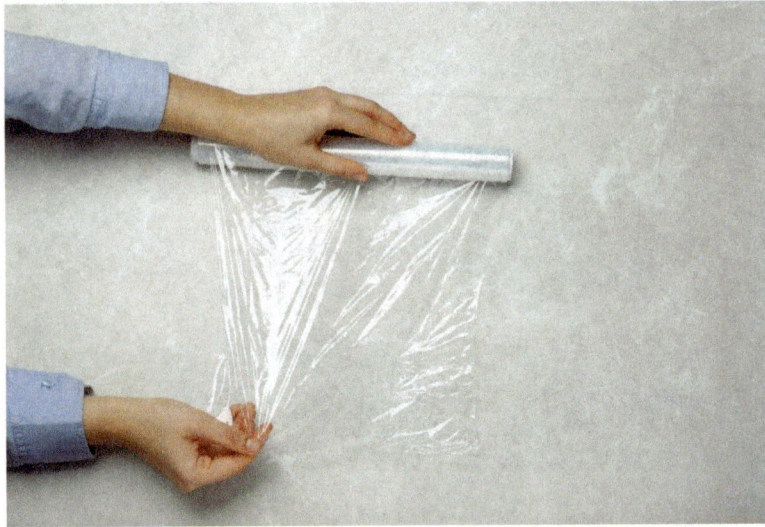

Chemicals
Ice-Frostbite
Dry-cooker
-fire
Eletricity
Radiation
Scald

Size
Cause-chemical
-electrical
Age
Location
Delth

ASTHMA

WHAT IS ASTHMA?

Asthma is a chronic inflammatory disease of the airway. During an asthmatic attack, the air passages of the lungs go into a spasm and, consequently, the airway narrows and the casualty begins to find it difficult to breathe.

CAUSES OF ASTHMA
- Allergies.
- Cold.
- Drugs.
- Cigarette smoke.

Whilst these factors may trigger an asthmatic attack, sometimes an attack can happen suddenly.

HOW TO RECOGNISE AN ASTHMA ATTACK

- Difficulty breathing.
- Wheezing.
- Difficulty speaking.
- Coughing.
- Distress and anxiety.
- Grey-blue tinge to the lips, earlobes, and nail beds (a condition known as cyanosis).
- Exhaustion.
- In severe cases, the casualty may lose consciousness.

TREATMENT OF ASTHMA — THE INHALER

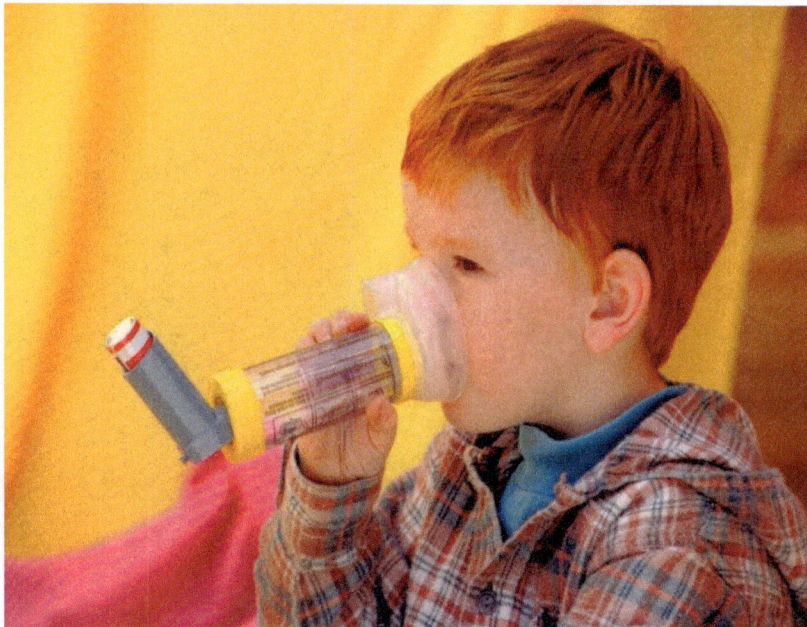

WHEN TO CALL AN AMBULANCE

If the asthma attack is:

- Happening for the first time.
- The attack is severe.
- The medication has no effect.
- They become exhausted.

ANAPHYLAXIS

Anaphylaxis is a severe abnormal allergic reaction of the body's immune system to a trigger.

When the casualty encounters a trigger, the immune system reacts by producing substantial amounts of histamine, which leads to reactions on the skin, airway, and circulation.

The list in the next slide can cause fatal anaphylactic reactions. The triggers are not limited to the ones listed below. If in any doubt, please seek medical assistance.

RECOGNISING ANAPHYLAXIS
- Blotchy skin rash.
- Red, watery, itchy eyes.
- Swollen hands, feet, and face.
- Stomach pain, vomiting, and diarrhoea.
- Minor to severe difficulty breathing.
- Pale and flushing skin.
- Swollen airway and throat. The tongue may also swell, and the eyes might appear puffy.
- A drop in blood pressure resulting from the widening of the blood vessels.

TRIGGERS OF ANAPHYLAXIS

FOOD-
The following foods have been identified as triggers for severe allergic reactions:

Milk, fish, chickpeas, crustaceans, bananas, snails, yeast, sherbet, nectarines, grapes, strawberries.

NUTS:
Peanut.
Walnut.
Almond.
Brazil.
Hazel.

DRUGS AND MEDICINES

ANTIBIOTICS
- Penicillin.
- Cephalosporin.
- Amphotericin.
- Ciprofloxacin.
- Vancomycin.

OTHER DRUGS
Gelatines.
Local Anaesthetics.

TREATMENT

Call 999/112

If the casualty is feeling faint and dizzy, lay them down and elevate their legs.

If the casualty is only finding it difficult to breathe, get them to sit up but continue to monitor them for dizziness and fainting.

If the casualty has an autoinjector, help them to use it. If they cannot administer it and you have the training to do so, then you may give it to them.

Pull off the safety cap, hold the autoinjector 10 cm away from the casualty, and press the tip against the outer part of the casualty's thigh until you can hear the click. Leave it in place for 10 seconds and then remove it. Massage the area for 10 seconds.

Let them sit up if they are experiencing breathing difficulties, and if feeling pale and faint, lay them down with their legs elevated.

SHOCK

Shock occurs when there is a failure of the circulatory system (heart, blood, and blood vessels) caused by a fall in blood pressure and blood volume. When this happens, the tissues of the body are starved of oxygen.

RECOGNITION OF SHOCK
- Pale, clammy skin.
- As the shock gets worse, the colour of the casualty's skin changes to grey-blue.
- Dizziness.
- Rapid breathing, and then shallow breathing.
- Fast pulse; slow pulse.
- Sweating.
- Weakness.
- Restlessness and aggressiveness; gasping for air; nausea, vomiting, and thirst.

TREATMENT OF SHOCK

TREATMENT OF SHOCK CONTINUED

Lie the casualty down with their back on the floor and their legs elevated above the level of their heart. The aim of this treatment is to improve the flow of blood to the brain.

Call 999/112 for emergency help, informing the emergency services that you suspect shock.
Loosen any tight clothing.
Keep the casualty warm.
Advise the casualty not to move.
Monitor and record their vital signs.

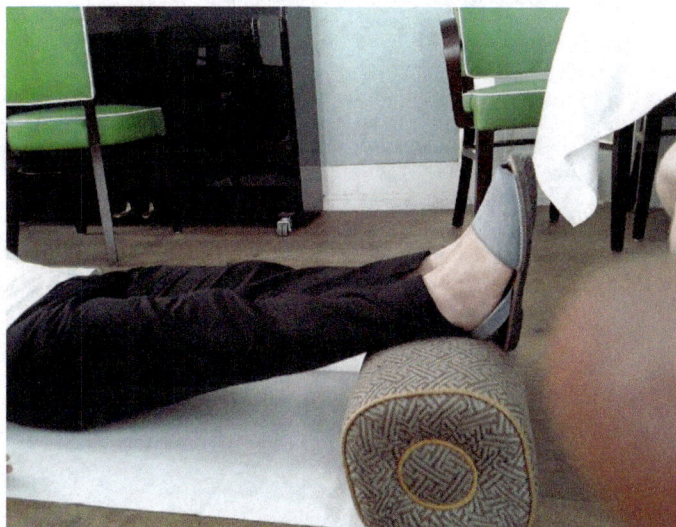

FAINTING

A faint occurs when a person suffers a brief loss of consciousness triggered by a temporary reduction of blood to the brain.

CAUSES OF FAINTING
- Pain.
- Exhaustion.
- Hunger.
- Emotional stress.
- A prolonged period of standing/sitting still leads to blood pooling in the legs and reduced blood to the brain.

RECOGNITION OF FAINTING
Initially slow pulse rate and then the pulse rate picks up and normalises.
The casualty loses consciousness briefly and collapses to the floor.
Pale, cold, and sweating.

TREATMENT POSITION FOR FAINTING
Lie the casualty down with their back on the floor and their legs elevated. The aim of this treatment is to improve the flow of blood to the brain.

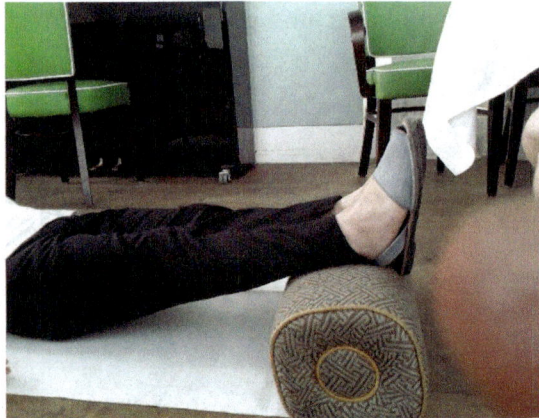

After 15 minutes of rest, the casualty should be able to conduct his or her work.

Dehydration

When the body loses fluid, it must be replaced sufficiently, otherwise, this can lead to dehydration.

A person can begin to dehydrate when he loses as much as one percent of his body weight. As the body loses fluid, it also loses minerals. An average person needs to drink an average of 2.5 litres (4 pints of water) daily.

Causes of dehydration:
- Excessive sweating due to playing sports.
- Exposure to the sun for prolonged periods.
- Fever.
- Diarrhoea.
- Vomiting.

WHO IS VULNERABLE TO DEHYDRATION?

- Young people.
- Elderly.
- Prolonged physical activity.

Recognition
- Dry mouth.
- Dry eyes.
- Dry/cracked lips.
- Headaches.
- Dark urine.
- Infrequent urination/reduction in amount of urine passed.
- Cramps.

DISLOCATION

Dislocation is the partial or full displacement of the bone from a joint.

Parts of the body you can dislocate
- Pelvis.
- Collar bone.
- Jaw.
- Knee.
- Elbow.

Common causes of dislocation
- Forceful impact.
- Unnatural movement.
- Sporting accidents.

Recognition of dislocation

- Pain.
- Swelling.
- Loss of power/movement.
- Deformity.
- Difficulty moving.

TREATMENT OF DISLOCATION

- Support with a sling.
- Do not put the bone back in.
- Take or send the casualty to hospital.
- Treat them for shock.

Improvised treatment for dislocation

If a casualty dislocates an elbow, it is usually a triangular bandage that is used to support the elbow. However, a sling will not always be available. If that is the case, then use any cloth you can find, even the casualty's own piece of clothing.

ARM SLING

The arm sling provides support for an injured upper arm, wrist or forearm and helps to support the arm where there is a rib fracture.

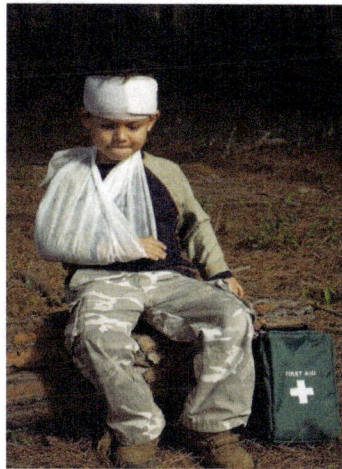

ELEVATED SLINGS

This elevated sling is used to support the arm if the patient injures his hand. It helps to control bleeding in the forearm or hand and reduces to the hand or forearm.

Step 1
Ask the patient to sit down and support the affected arm across their chest ensuring that the fingers rest on the opposite shoulder.

Step 2
The bandage should be placed across the patient's shoulder with on the uninjured side. Hold the point of the bandage beyond the elbow on the injured arm.

Step 3
Tuck the bandage under the patient's hand , forearm, and elbow.

Step 4
The lower end of the bandage should be linked up diagonally across the back with the other end at the patient's shoulder.

Step 5
Tie a knot where both ends meet

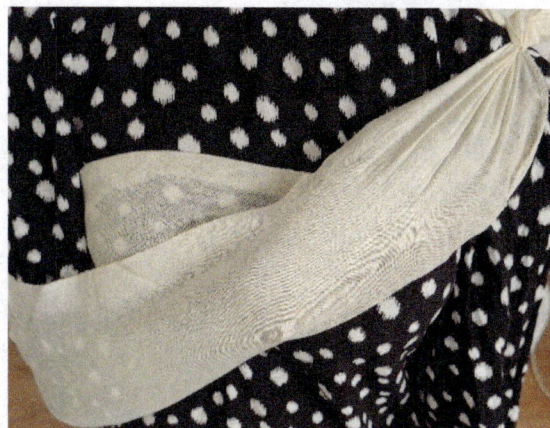

How to use the casualty's own jacket to make a sling.

Step 1 – Unbutton the jacket without removing it.
Step 2 – Fold the lower edge of the injured side over the injured arm.
Step 3 – Secure the hem of the jacket breast, feeding it with a large safety pin.
Step 4 – Tuck and pin any excess material around the casualty's elbow.

FRACTURE

A fracture is a break in the continuity of the bones.

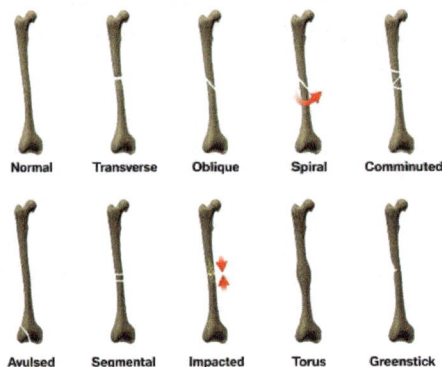

Treatment of an open fracture

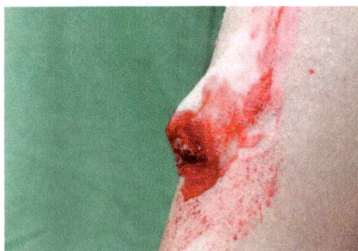

Any fracture where the skin is damaged is an open fracture. A bone might be seen protruding from the skin but not necessarily in all cases.
An appropriate treatment is to control any bleeding by applying pressure around the injury but ensuring that no pressure is placed on the injury itself.

Do not move the limb—leave it in the position found.

Call 999/112.

Look out for signs of shock and treat accordingly.

CLOSED FRACTURE

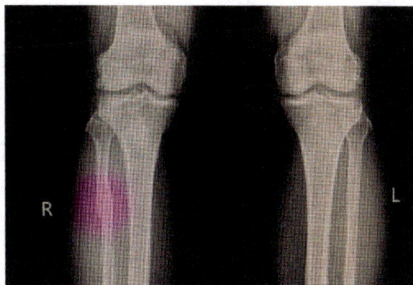

Spinal Injury

A spinal injury can lead to paralysis or death of the casualty if the spinal cord is damaged.
The spine protects nerves that are responsible for controlling movement and breathing.
The provision of immediate medical care can make the difference between life or death and can determine the extent of the casualty.

Consequences of a spinal cord injury
- Loss of power.
- Loss of sensation.
- Complete severing of the spinal cord can lead to irreparable damage to the casualty.

Causes of spinal injury
The severity of a spinal injury depends on how it happened.

The factors to consider are:
- Was excessive force applied to the neck/back?
- Did the casualty bend forward or backward forcefully?
- Did the casualty twist the spine?

Other causes

- Falling from height.
- Car accident.
- Diving into a shallow swimming pool.
- Falling from a horse.
- Collapsed rugby scrum.
- Injury to the head.

Recognising a spinal injury

- Pain in the neck/back.
- Lack of movement in the limb.
- Lack of sensation or tingling sensation in the limbs.
- Loss of bowel or bladder control.
- Tenderness of the skin or the spine.
- Awkward position of the head in relation to other parts of the body.
- Breathing difficulties.

Treatment of a conscious casualty who you suspect to have spinal injury
- Provide reassurance.
- Discourage any movement.
- You must immobilise their head and neck, ensuring the head and neck are aligned with the rest of the body.
- Call 999/112 for help.
- Keep the casualty warm and still.

Treating an unconscious casualty with a spinal injury
- If they are breathing normally, do not tilt their head back, just immobilise it.
- If the casualty is not breathing normally, you will have to tilt their head back and maintain the airway by using the jaw thrust.
- If you must leave the casualty to get help, then you should put him/her in the recovery position.
- If the casualty is not breathing, then commence CPR.
- Continue to monitor and record the casualty's vital signs.
- Call 999/112 for help.

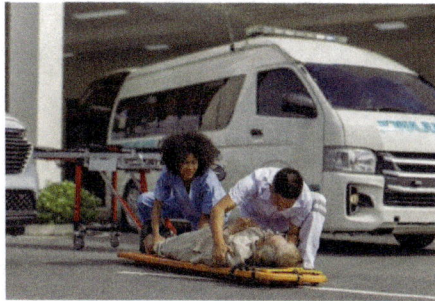

Forearm and Wrist Injuries

CAUSES OF FOREARM AND WRIST INJURIES
Fractures caused by direct impact on the forearm or wrist.
A fall on the arm can also cause an injury to the wrist or forearm.
Falling on an outstretched hand can result in wrist injuries.
The injury around the wrist is likely to be a sprain, but if in any doubt, always treat it as a fracture. If it is a sprained wrist, you can apply ice, but if you are in any doubt, just place the injured wrist in an arm sling.

RECOGNITION
- Pain.
- Swelling.
- Bruising.
- Deformity.
- Possible fracture.

TREATMENT

Get the casualty to sit down.
Place their injured forearm in an arm sling.
Put padding around the injured forearm and support with a triangular bandage.
Always tie any knots on the injured side.
Secure the art sling with a broad fold.

STRAINS AND SPRAINS

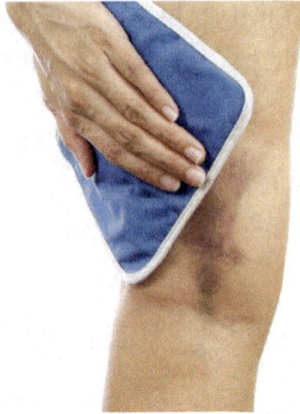

STRAIN – An injury to the muscles or to the tendon.

SPRAIN – An injury to the ligament.

Treatment

R – Rest.

I – Ice.

C – Comfortable support.

E – Elevate the injured part.

POISONING

A poison is any substance that when ingested, instilled, or absorbed into the body, can lead to permanent or temporary damage to the body.

Routes of entry of poison into the body:

- Inhalation.
- Instilled.
- Injected.
- Absorbed.

Signs and symptoms

Nausea.

Vomiting.

Abdominal pain.

Seizures.

Irregular heartbeat.

Varying levels of consciousness.

Difficulty breathing.

Hypoxia.

Swelling.

Anaphylactic shock.

Cyanosis.

Itching.

TREATMENT

- Call 999/112, call poison control, and follow their instructions.
- Commence CPR if required.
- Use a face mask to minimise the risk of infection.
- Remove contaminated clothing.
- If the poison is absorbed in the eyes, you must wash them for 10 minutes.
- If the injected poison is through a bee sting, then remove the sting by scraping it off with the edge of a credit card.
- If the poison is by way of inhalation, then help the casualty into the fresh air.

- If the patient has a chemical on their skin, then remove their clothing and wash the affected area for about 20 minutes.

HEAD INJURY

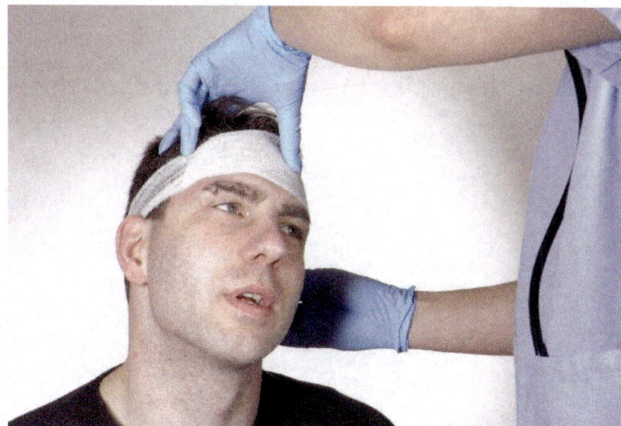

CAUSES OF A HEAD INJURY

- Falling.
- Blow to the head.
- Car accidents.

- The impact of falling from a height can transfer up the body and damage the base of the train.

TYPES OF HEAD INJURY

CONCUSSION
This is when the brain shakes because of a blow to the head.

Signs of concussion
- Temporary loss of consciousness.
- Confusion.
- Any sign of a scalp wound.
- Short memory loss.
- Mild headache.

COMPRESSION
This is when there is pressure on the brain caused by bleeding, or swelling of the brain caused by direct or indirect impact.

- Be mindful of patients with a history of head injuries.
- Deteriorating levels of consciousness.
- Loss of consciousness.
- Watch out for blood flowing from the ear or the patient's nose.

Management of a severe head injury:

- Call 999/112.
- Open the casualty's airway.
- Do not move the patient.
- If you suspect a spinal injury, then using the jaw thrust to open the airway is advisable.
- Monitor vital organs.

FRACTURE
This is caused by a skull fracture.

USING THE AVPU SCALE:

A – Is the patient alert? Are his eyes open, does he respond to your questions?
V – Does he respond to your voice.
P – Does he respond to a stimulus of pain?
U – If he does not respond to any stimulus, then he is deemed to be unresponsive.

Central Nervous System
(Brain)

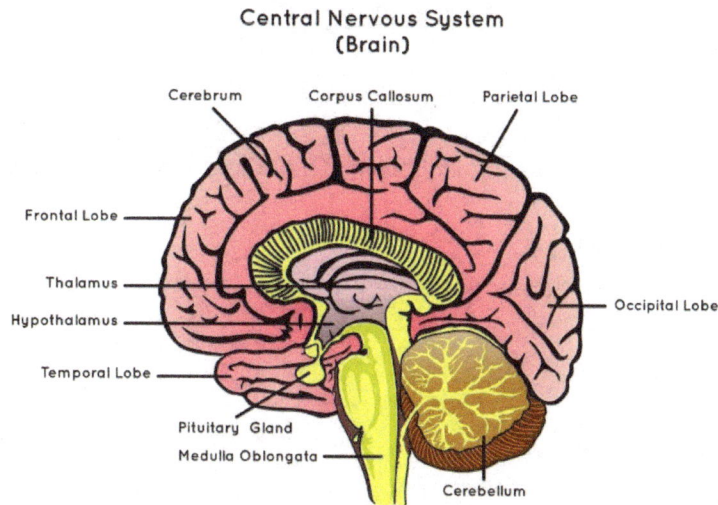

Cerebrum · Corpus Callosum · Parietal Lobe
Frontal Lobe
Thalamus
Hypothalamus
Occipital Lobe
Temporal Lobe
Pituitary Gland
Medulla Oblongata
Cerebellum

MANAGEMENT OF A HEAD INJURY

- Get the patient to sit down and provide a cold compress so the patient can hold it against the injury.

- Monitor the patient's vital organs by checking their breathing, pulse, and his level of response.

- Make sure the patient's recovery is monitored by a responsible person.

- Where the injury is the result of a sporting accident, do not allow the patient to return to the sport until a doctor has checked them.

- If he is worsening, then get the patient to seek medical assistance.

Signs of a worsening head injury:
- Drowsiness.
- Continuing headache.
- Confusion, dizziness, or loss of memory.
- Impaired speech.
- Impaired movement.
- Vomiting.
- Uneven pupil size.

MENINGITIS

What is meningitis?

This is an infection of the lining surrounding the brain. The lining is called the meninges.

Recognition
- Flu-like symptoms with associated high fever.
- Cold hands and feet.
- Pain in the casualty's joint door limb.
- Pale skin.
- Signs of worsening of the illness.
- Severe headache.
- Stiff neck.
- Vomiting.
- Aversion to bright light.
- Drowsiness.

Signs of meningitis in infants

- Bulging and hardening of the fontanelle.
- Crying with a high-pitched voice.

Final stages of the illness:

A rash on the skin, which does not disappear when pressed. Colour of the rash could be red or purple.

Treatment
Seek urgent medical help if you see any of the signs develop. Do not wait for all the signs and symptoms to appear.

Look out for a rash.

Provide reassurance.

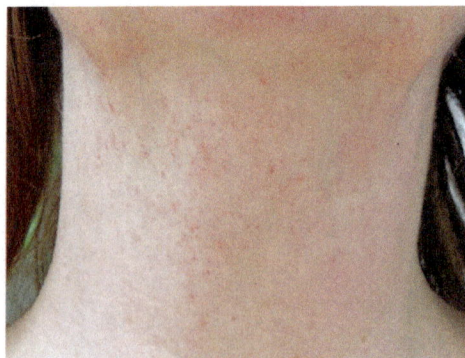

HYPOTHERMIA

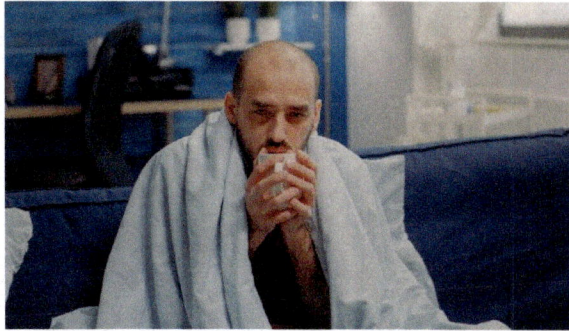

Hypothermia occurs when the body temperature falls below 35 degrees (95 degrees Fahrenheit).

Moderate Hypothermia is Reversible

SEVERE HYPOTHERMIA occurs when the core body temperature falls below 30 degrees. This is often but not always fatal. Do not discontinue lifesaving procedures until emergency help arrives.

CAUSES OF HYPOTHERMIA
Exposure to cold over a prolonged period.
Immersion in freezing water.
Poorly heated/insulated homes.

THOSE VULNERABLE TO HYPOTHERMIA
- Old people.
- Infants.
- Frail people.
- Think people.
- Inactivity.
- Chronic illnesses.
- Fatigue.

Alcohol and drugs can make this worse.

RECOGNITION
- Shivering.
- Cold, pale, and dry skin.
- Apathy.
- Irrational behaviour.
- Disorientation.
- Lethargy and impaired consciousness.
- Slow and shallow breathing.
- Slow, weak pulse.

TREATMENT WHEN OUTDOORS

- Move the casualty from the cold to a sheltered place.
- Do not lay casualty on a bare ground—preferably lay on an insulating material (e.g., pine branches).
- Cover with a blanket and then wrap in a foil serving bag or plastic. Your body can provide further heat.
- Remove all wet clothing.
- Cover his head.
- Call 999/112.

GUIDELINES ON CALLING FOR HELP IN REMOTE AREAS

- Two people should go for help.
- Do not leave the casualty on his own.
- For a responsive casualty, give warm drinks/give chocolates if any.
- Monitor the casualty's vital signs before help arrives.

TREATMENT WHEN INDOORS

- Warm casualty with blankets.
- Give warm drinks, e.g. soup/chocolate.
- Seek medical advice.
- Monitor vital signs.

HYPOTHERMIA IN INFANTS

WHY WOULD AN INFANT SUFFER FROM HYPOTHERMIA?

The thermostat in the baby's brain, which regulates temperature, is not as fully developed as it is with adults.

RECOGNITION OF HYPOTHERMIA IN INFANTS

- Skin may be cold.
- Baby may be limp.
- Unusually quiet.
- Refusing to feed.

TREATMENT OF INFANTS SUFFERING FROM HYPOTHERMIA

- Warm the baby with a blanket.
- Warm the room.
- Seek medical advice.

HEATSTROKE

This occurs when there is a failure of the part of the brain that regulates temperature. That part of the brain is called the hypothalamus. When heat stroke occurs, the body temperature increases to intolerable levels.

CAUSES OF HEATSTROKE

- High fever.
- Exposure to heat over a prolonged period.
- Taking certain types of drugs like ecstasy can cause overheating of the body.
- Heat exhaustion when the casualty is no longer sweating, making it impossible for the body to be cooled by evaporating sweat.

RECOGNITION

- Headache.
- Dizziness.
- Restlessness and confusion.
- Hot, flushed dry skin.
- A rapid deterioration of the level of consciousness.
- Full bounding pulse.
- Body temperature rises above 40 degrees.

TREATMENT

- Move the casualty to a cool place.

- Remove clothing where possible.

- Call 999/112.

- Sit the casualty down and provide support behind them.

- Wrap a cold, wet sheet over the casualty until the temperature falls to 38°C (100.4F) (under the tongue) or 37.5°C (99.5F) under the armpit.

- Continue to pour water over the sheet wrapped over the casualty.

- In the absence of a sheet, just fan or sponge the casualty with chilly water.

- Continue to cool the casualty until the casualty returns to normal.

- Once the casualty returns to normal, change the wet sheets and wrap him in dry ones.

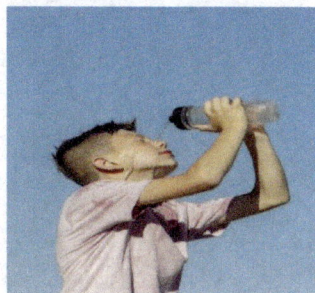

UNRESPONSIVE, NON-BREATHING CHILD

CHECK FOR DANGER

Always assess the environment to ensure you are safe and the child is not exposed to any further harm. If you see danger, make sure the area is safe or move the child away from danger and commence immediate treatment.

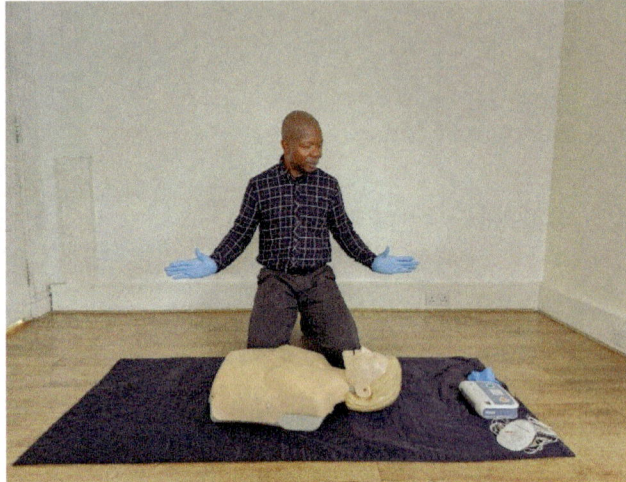

Check for responsiveness.

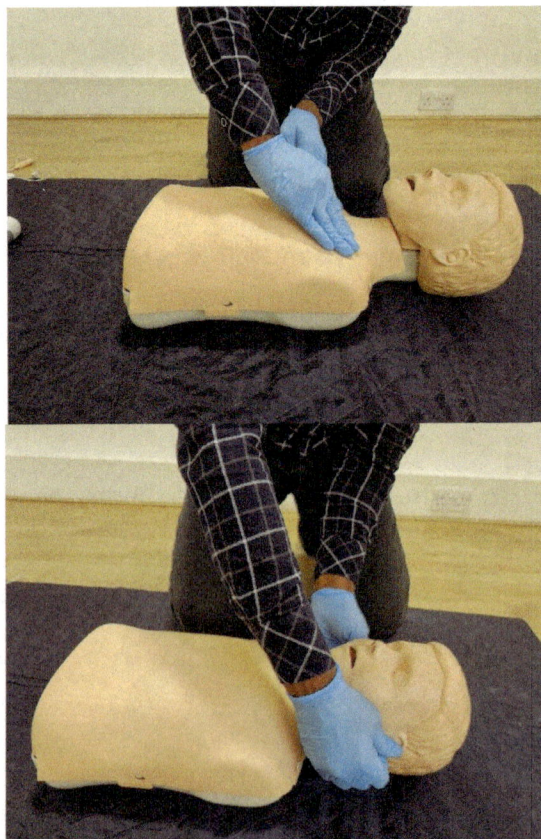

Talk to the child. Ask, "What happened?"
Give a command, "Open your eyes."
Tap the shoulder for a response.

Check the Airway

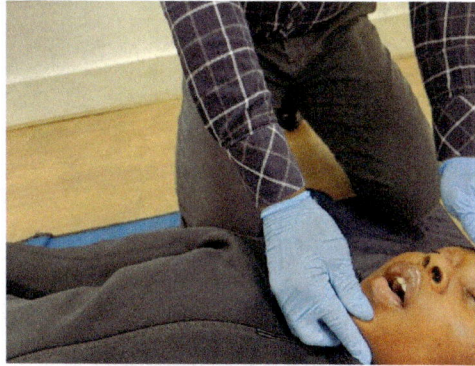

IF THE CHILD IS RESPONSIVE

Follow the primary survey: DR ABC

Treat the injuries—worst injuries first.

Check breathing, pulse, and how the casualty is responding until emergency help arrives or he gets better.

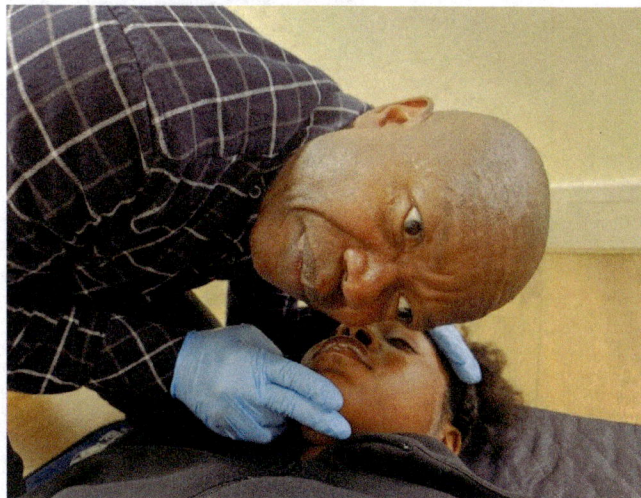

Child Rescue Breath: Squeeze the nose and open the mouth with a face shield.

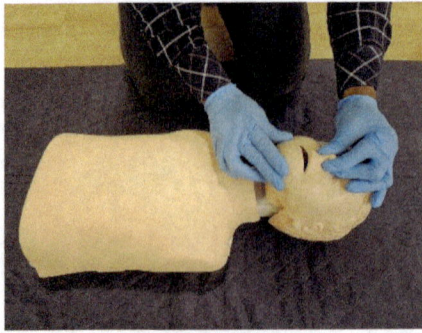

Child CPR
Rescue Breath: Mouth-to-Mouth

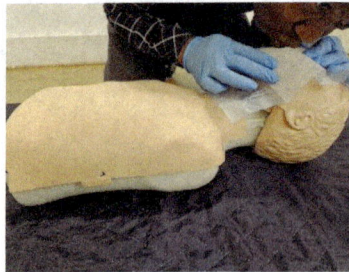

Child Rescue Breath: Mouth to pocket mask

Five rescue breaths and 30 compressions followed by two rescue breaths. After the first rescue breaths, the subsequent rescue breaths should be two and then 30 chest compressions until the patient recovers.

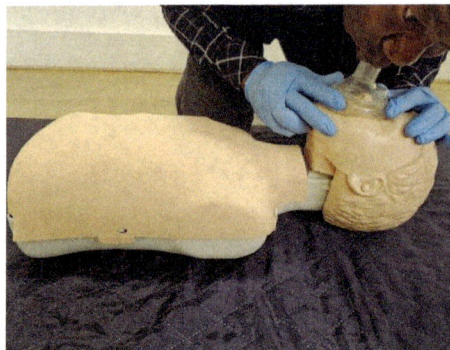

Child Compressions
Child CPR: Defibrillating a child—back placement.

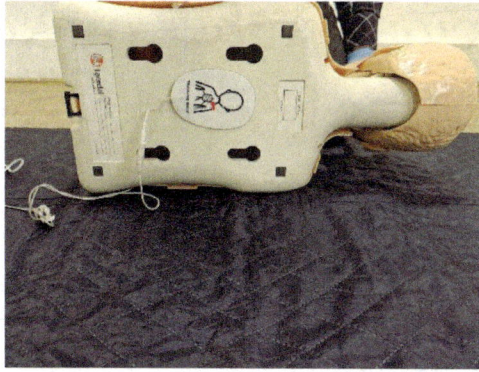

Child Chest compressions

Place the heel of your hand in the centre of the chest and give 30 chest compressions. Use one hand only unless you are dealing with a bigger child, in which case, you can use two hands.

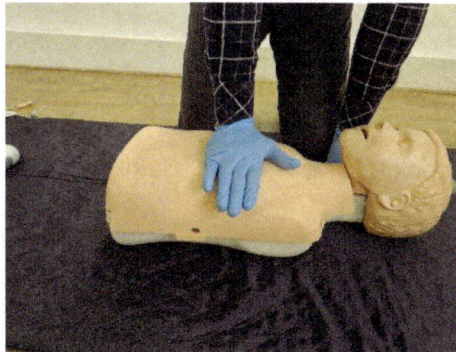

UNCONSCIOUS AND BREATHING ADULT

IF THE ADULT IS NOT RESPONSIVE:
- Shout for help
- Do not move him; leave him where was found and proceed to open his airway.

TO OPEN THE AIRWAY, FOLLOW THE FOLLOWING STEPS:

Look, listen and feel

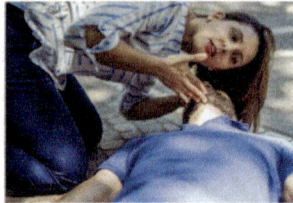

Place one hand on the forehead.

Place two fingers on the point of the chin, not the soft tissues on the chin to avoid blocking the airway, and tilt the head back slightly.

Look, hear, and feel for breathing.
HOW TO CHECK FOR BREATHING

Lean towards the head of the casualty with your cheek close to the casualty's nose.

Look: Is the adult's chest moving?

Listen: Can you hear the adult breathing normally?

Feel: Can you feel the adult's breathing on your cheek?

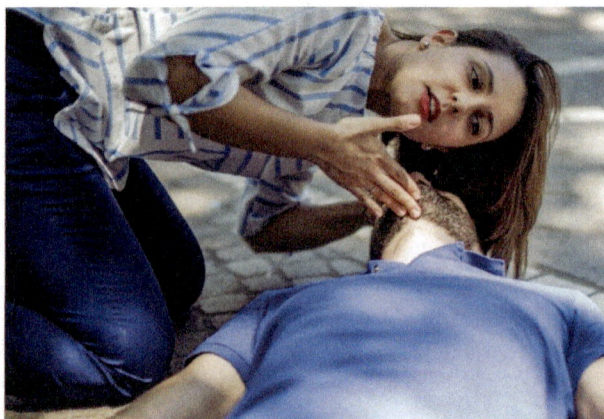

UNCONSCIOUS AND BREATHING ADULT

IS THE CASUALTY BREATHING?

Follow the primary survey, DR ABC. Treat serious conditions first.
Place the casualty on their side in the recovery position.

Recovery position:
- A safe and comfortable position aimed at opening the airway.
- Place the patient in a lateral position when unresponsive and breathing.
- Kneel beside the patient and straighten both legs.
- Place the arm nearest to you at a right angle to his body with his palm open.
- Bring the arm of the patient that is furthest away from you and place it on the cheek nearest to you and hold it there.
- Whilst holding the patient's hand to their cheek, raise the leg furthest from you with your hand on their knee and roll them over towards you. Ensure the patient's head is tilted and adjust his hip and leg so that they are bent and at the right angles.

Recovery Position

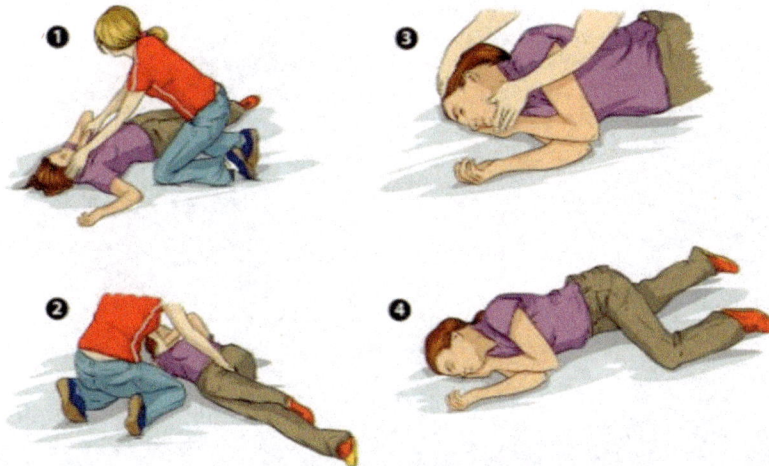

Call 999/112 for emergency help.

Check breathing, pulse, and the casualty's level of response until emergency help arrives.

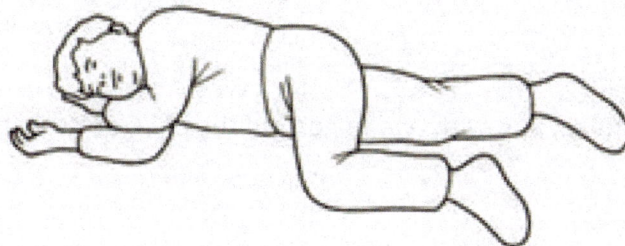

UNCONSCIOUS AND BREATHING CHILD

HOW TO PLACE A CHILD IN THE RECOVERY POSITION

Step 1
Kneel beside the casualty.

Step 2

Check for danger.

Make sure you are safe and the patient is also safe.

Step 3

Check if the patient is responsive to a stimulus of pain by squeezing their earlobes.

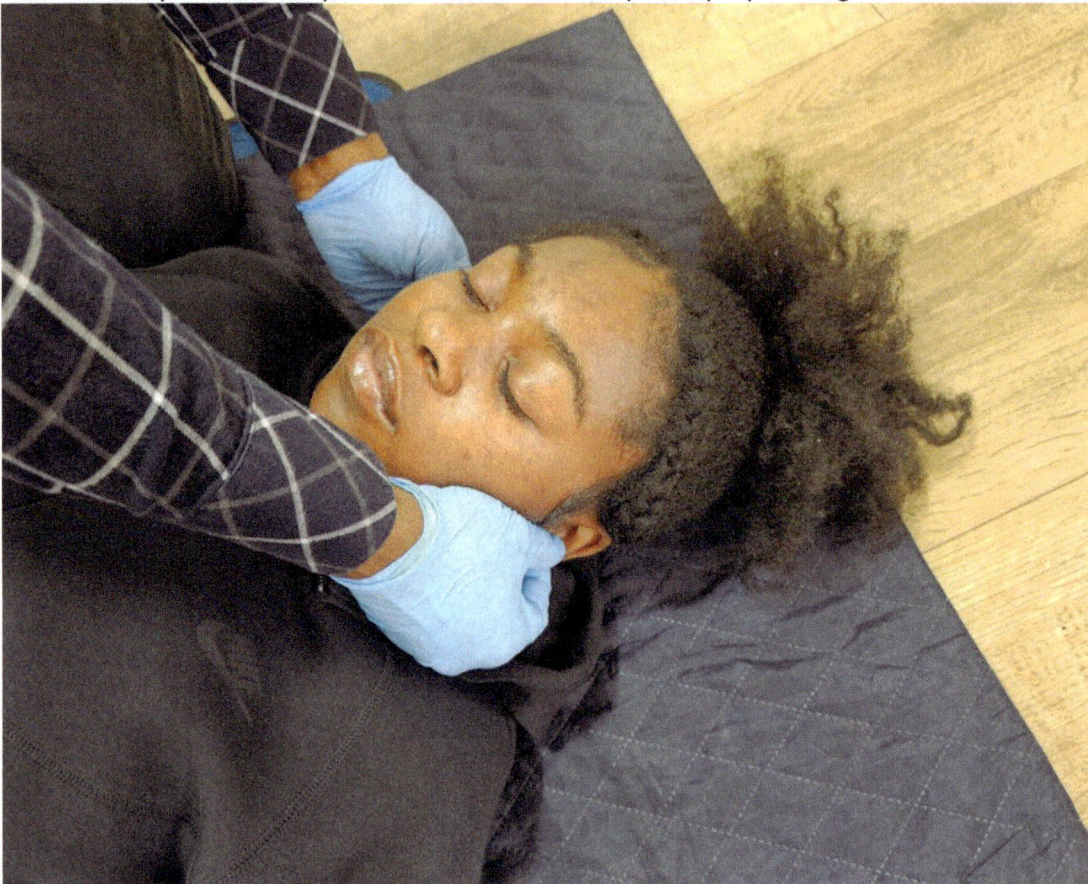

Step 4
Do a head tilt and chin lift.

Place one hand on the forehead, and with two fingers on the chin, do a head tilt and a chin lift.

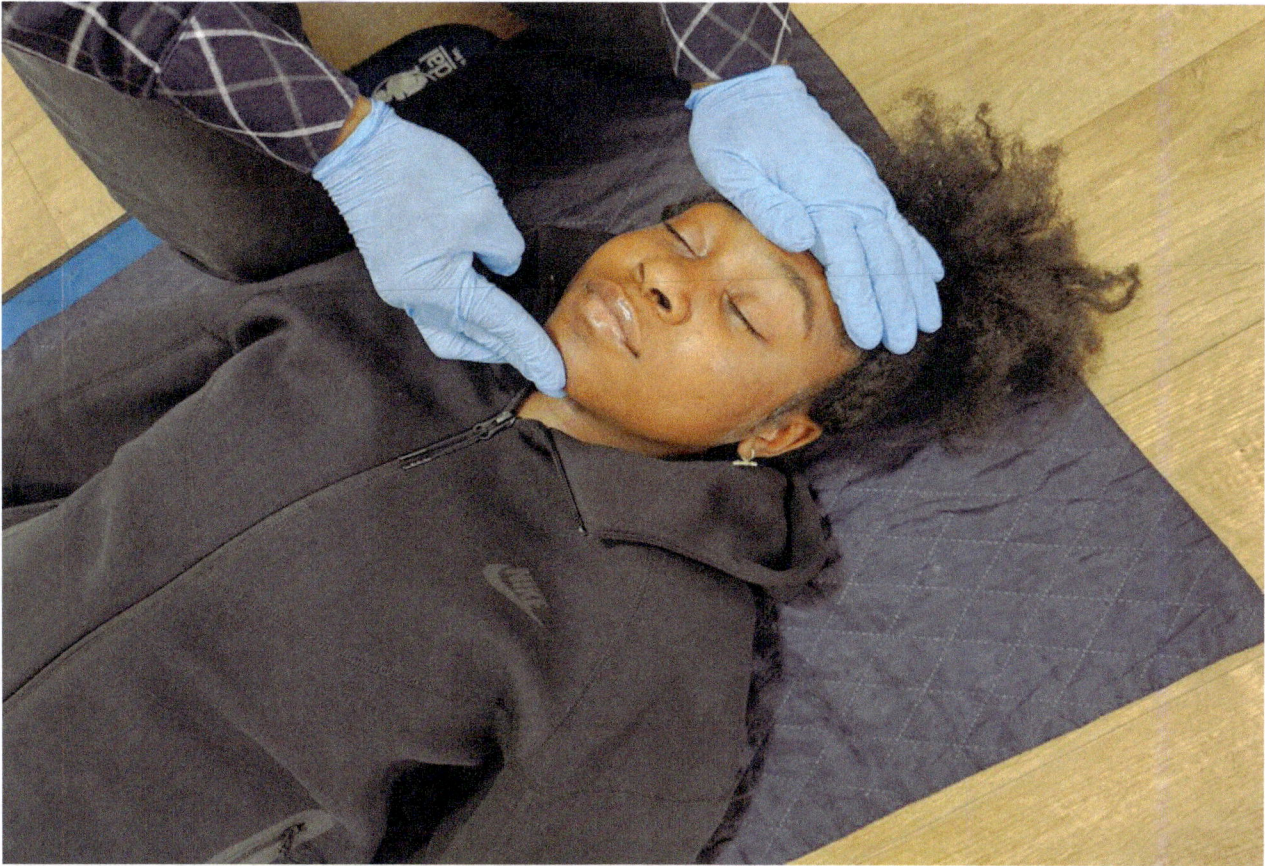

Step 5

Check if the child is breathing.

Lean towards the head with your cheek facing the casualty's nose to feel for the child's breath.

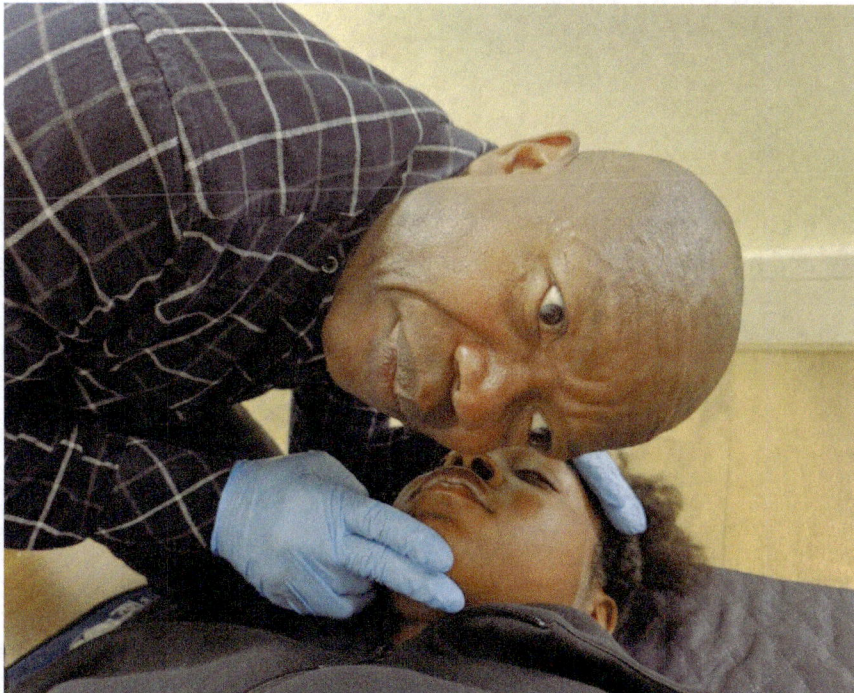

Step 6

Reach for the casualty's hand nearest to you and put it in a right-angled position or straight.

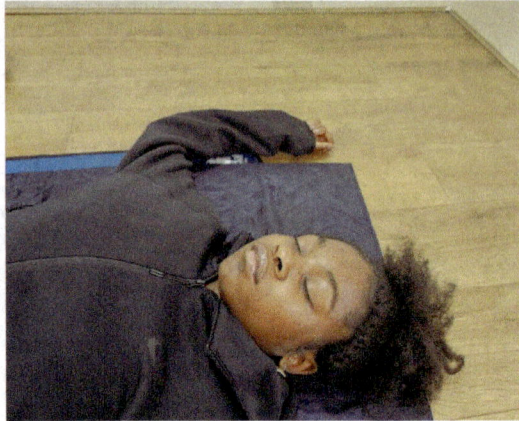

Step 7

reach out for the casualty's hand furthest from you and place it on his/her cheek and hold it there.

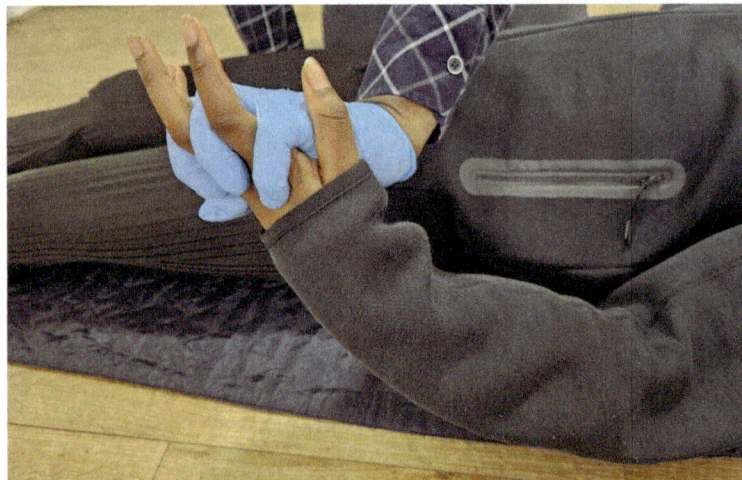

Step 8
Reach out for the child's arm furthest from you across his chest and place the back of his hand on the cheek nearest to you and hold it there, palm to palm.

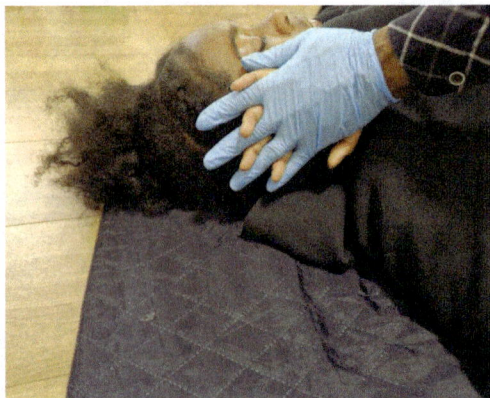

Step 9

Check the pockets for any sharp objects likely to cause harm to the patient. Check for bulky items in his pockets and remove any glasses.
Straighten the casualty's legs.

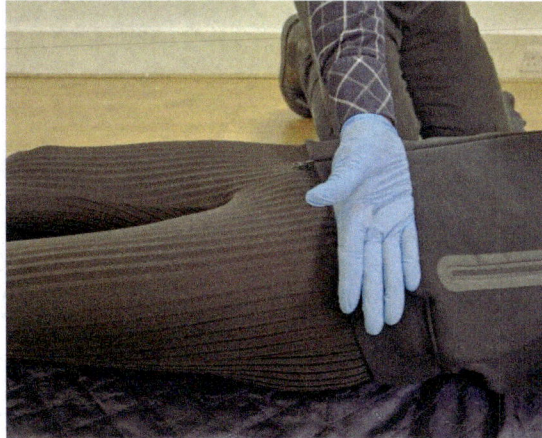

Step 10

Place the outer part of the child's leg that is furthest away from you around the knee.

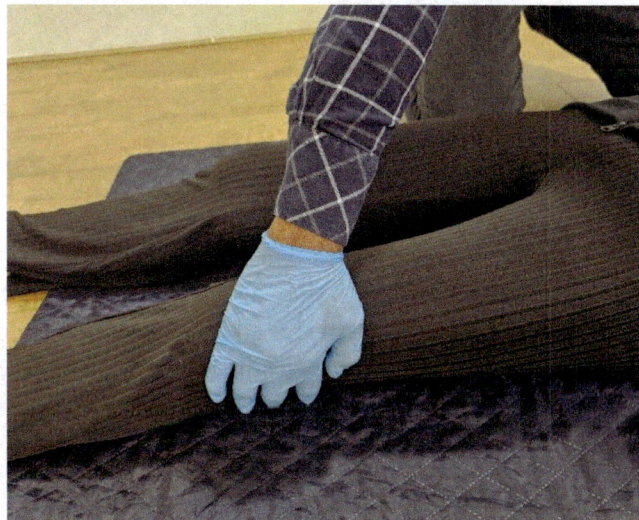

Step 11

Lift it up with your hand on top of the child's knee.

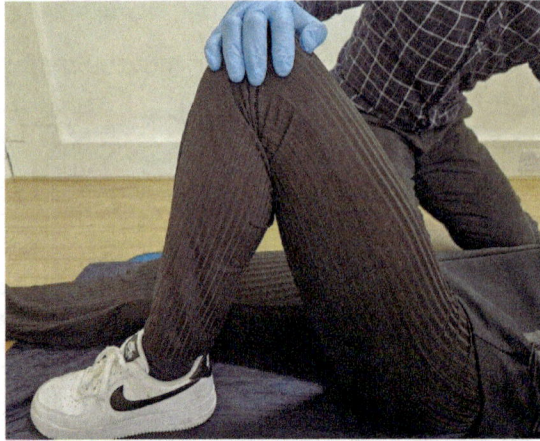

Step 12

Using the knee as a lever, roll the child on their side in a recovery position. Roll the child towards you.

Tilt the head back carefully to maintain a clear airway.

Check every minute to confirm the child is still breathing whilst waiting for an ambulance to arrive.

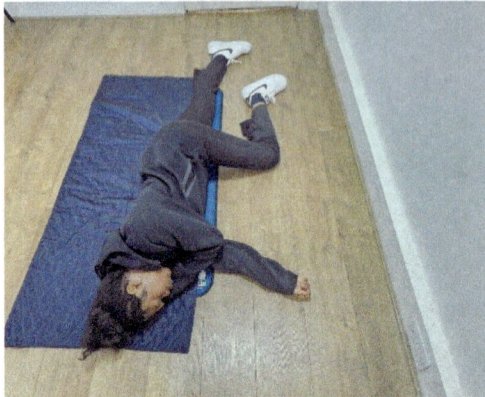

Reach for the leg furthest from you and raise the outer part of the child's leg with your hand placed on their knee, making sure the child's feet are firmly on the ground. Roll the child towards you. Adjust the upper leg so that the hip and knee are at right angles to the body. Again, tilt the chin up to clear the casualty's airway.

UNCONSCIOUS AND BREATHING INFANT

CHECK FOR A RESPONSE

Tap the sole of the infant's foot and talk to them as you do so to check for a response. Never shake the infant's shoulder.

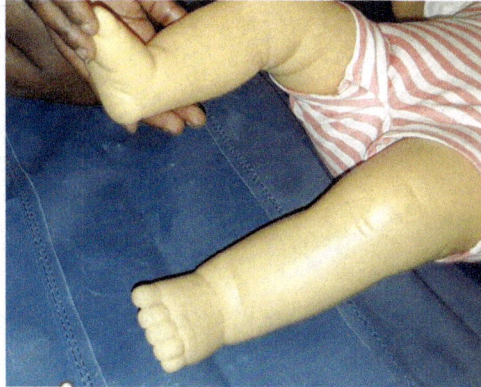

IF THE INFANT RESPONDS
Conduct the primary survey, DR ABC. Treat life-threatening injuries first.
Call for help if necessary.

IF THE INFANT DOES NOT RESPOND

Call for help.

Lay the baby on a flat and firm surface.

Open and check their airway.

HOW TO OPEN THE BABY'S AIRWAY
Place one hand on the forehead and tilt the head back.
Maintain the head tilt with a finger on the chin.

Check airway: head tilt, chin lift.

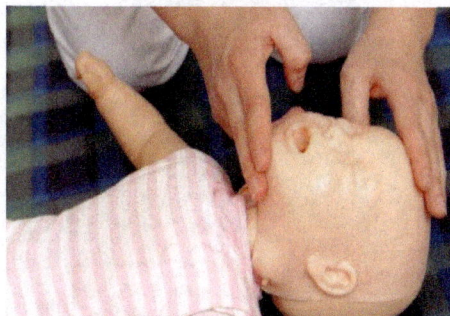

Check breathing: Look, listen, and feel.

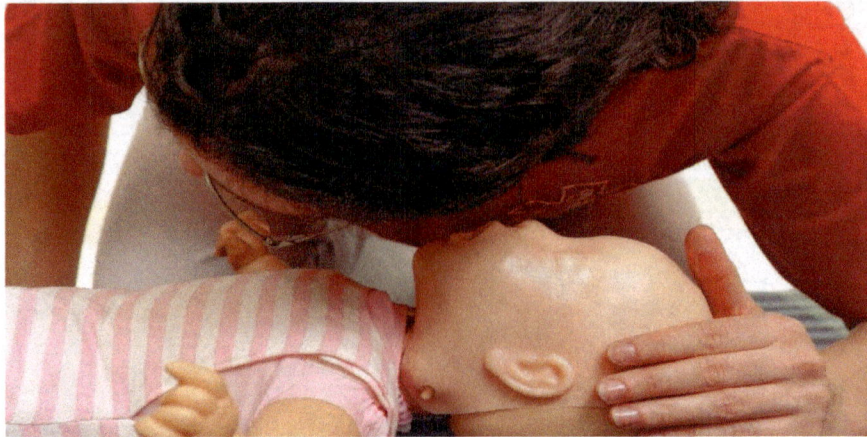

Avoid pressure on the soft part of the chin to prevent blockage of the infant's airway.

Check if the baby is breathing by bringing your head down to the baby's face so you can feel for breathing.

What do you do if the infant is breathing?
Once you confirm the infant is breathing, conduct a primary survey—DR ABC

Put the baby in the recovery position by cuddling them in your arms with the head of the baby lower than the bottom to clear the airway.
Continue to monitor breathing and the baby's pulse if you have the skills to check the pulse.

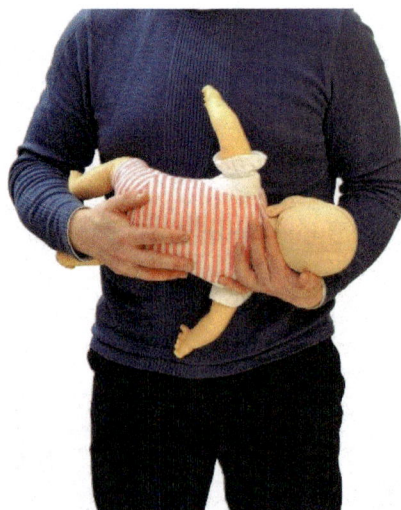

UNCONSCIOUS AND NON-BREATHING BABY

If the baby is not breathing, call 999/112 for emergency help.

Perform CPR for one minute before calling for help.

If you have a phone, then put the phone's speaker on and call 999/112 for emergency help. If the phone is not with you, take the baby with you to make the emergency phone call.

Conduct CPR.

Give five rescue breaths to start with.

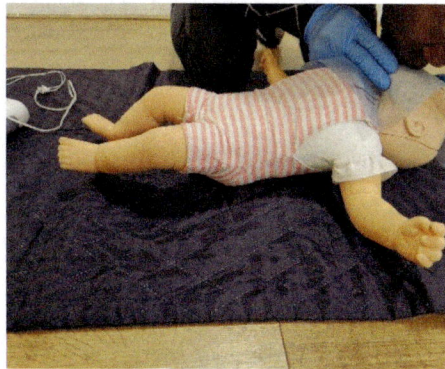

Followed by 30 chest compressions.

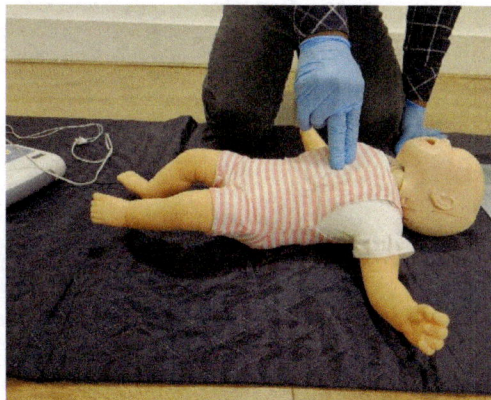

And then give another two rescue breaths. All subsequent rescue breathing must be two followed by 30 chest compressions.

START CPR IF THE CASUALTY SUFFERS FROM A CARDIAC ARREST

CPR stands for cardiopulmonary resuscitation. This is a combination of rescue breaths (mouth-to-mouth, nose-to-mouth, or mouth-to-stoma) and compression on the chest of the casualty.

Check that the casualty is responsive. Shake their shoulders and raise your voice close to the casualty's ears. Talk to them. Give a command, "Open your eyes." If the casualty is not responding, then call for help.

UNCONSCIOUS AND NON-BREATHING ADULT

Kneel next to the casualty.

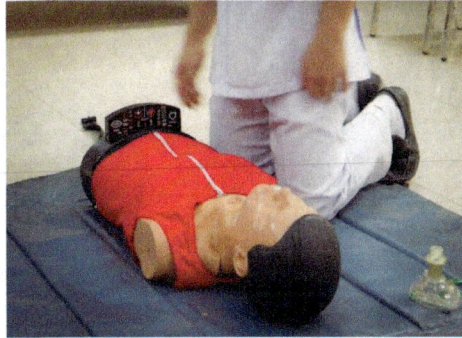

Check if the patient is responsive.

Check if the casualty is responsive by shouting their name and giving a verbal command such as "Open your eyes!" If they are not responding to your verbal command, tap on their shoulder. If they are still not responding, you can assume they are unresponsive.

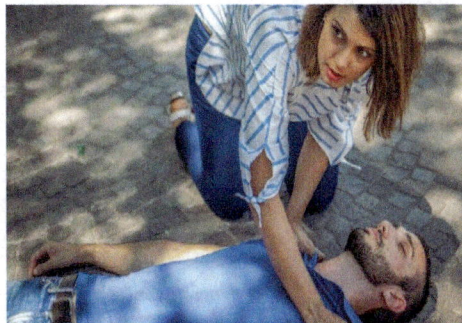

Open the patient's airway.

Open the casualty's airway by conducting a head tilt chin lift. You place one hand on the patient's forehead and use two fingers to lift his chin up. Pinch the casualty's nose with the same hand on the forehead. Make sure you are only pinching the soft part of the nose with a finger and thumb. The casualty's mouth should open when you squeeze the nose and tilt the head back.

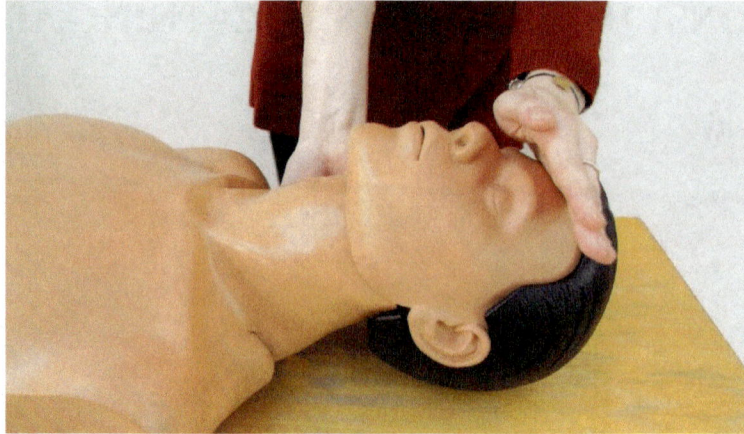

Check if the patient is breathing. Check for 10 seconds.

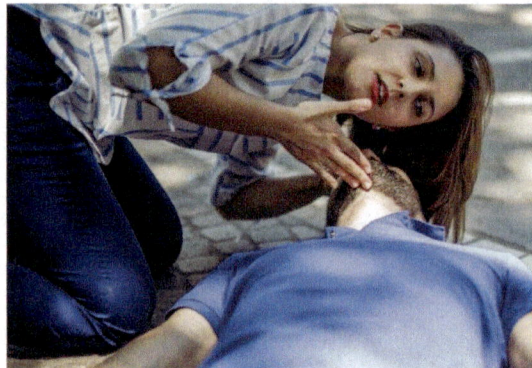

If the casualty is not breathing, call 999/112 for emergency help.

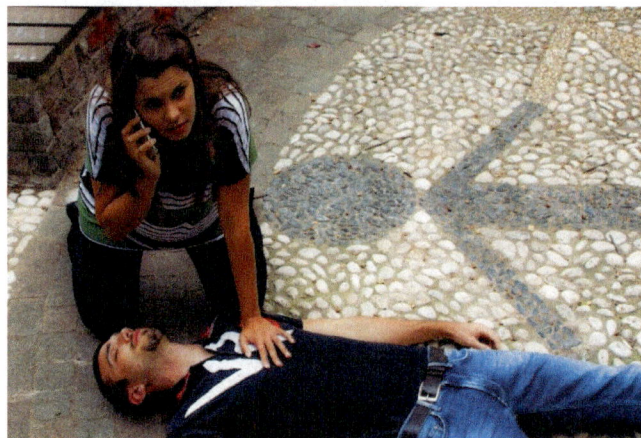

If you have a phone and you are on your own, then put the phone's speaker on and call 999/112 for emergency help.

If the phone is not with you and you must call for help, then do so first before commencing CPR.

START CHEST COMPRESSIONS
Place the heel of your hand in the centre of the casualty's chest, slightly above the tip of the breastbone. Place the second hand on top of the first hand, which is already positioned on the chest. Interlock your fingers and give 30 compressions at a rate of 100-120 compressions per minute.

Make sure your hands are straight and leaning slightly over the casualty.
Press down on the casualty's chest to a depth of 5-6 cm (2-2 ½ inches).

Release your pressure on the chest and watch it recoil before pressing down on it again.
The hand position is vital to the performance of effective CPR.

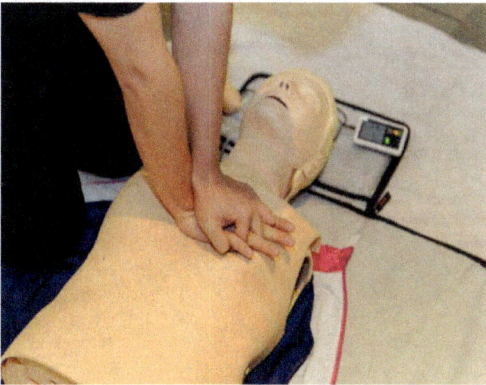

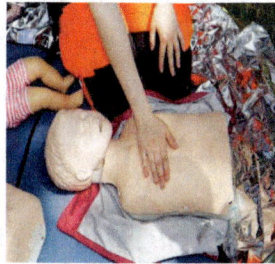

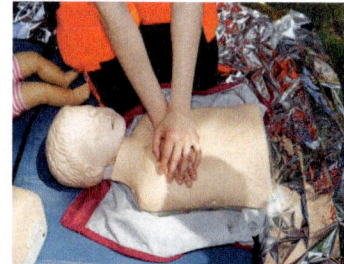

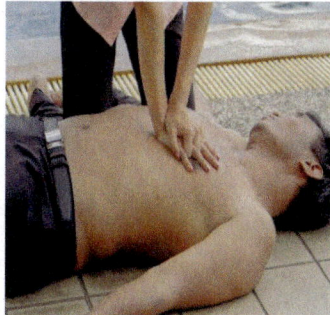

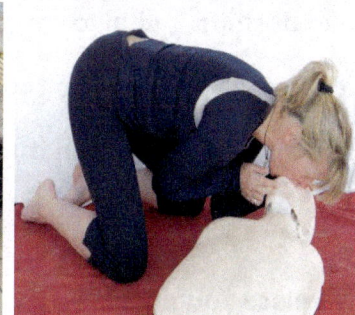

WHERE NOT TO PLACE YOUR HAND WHEN PERFORMING CPR:
- Avoid placing your hand on the ribs.
- Avoid placing your hand on the abdomen.
- Avoid placing your hand on the tip of the breastbone. Position your hands above the tip of the breastbone.

PERFORMING ADULT RESCUE BREATHS
Seal your lips tightly over the casualty's mouth and blow air into the casualty's mouth. You should see the casualty's chest rise.
The rescue breath should last no more than a minute.

If their chest does not rise, it might be because their head is not properly tilted back. Recheck and try again.

Maintain the head tilt, remove your mouth from the casualty's and watch their chest fall and then repeat the rescue breath.

Continue the rescue breath until the emergency services arrive.

If you are unable to conduct a rescue breath, then give continuous compressions. A rescuer may not want to give rescue breaths because they suspect the patient has an infection or has vomited, in those circumstances, continuous compressions can be administered to the patient until the emergency services arrive.

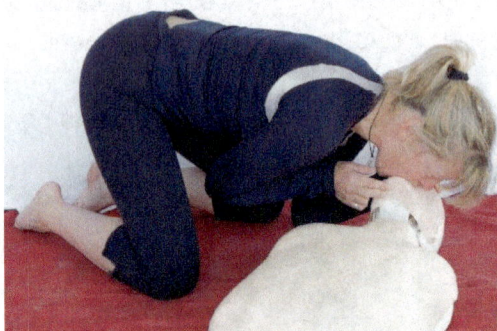

WHERE NOT TO PLACE YOUR HAND WHEN PERFORMING CPR

The hand position is vital to the performance of effective CPR.

• **Avoid placing your hand on the ribs.**

• **Avoid placing your hand on the abdomen.**

Don't place your hands on the ribs.

Don't place your hands on the abdomen.

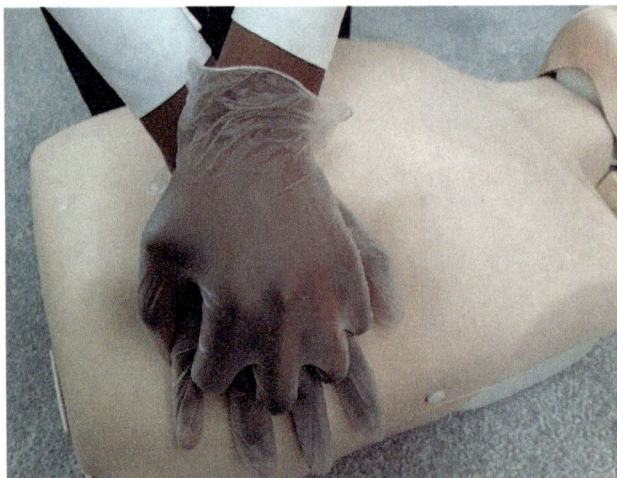

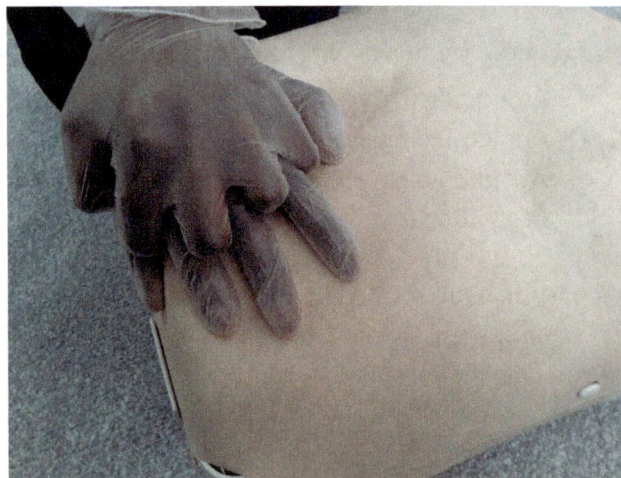

OBSTACLES TO DELIVERING EFFECTIVE CPR

Your role as a first aider or first responder is to minimize the risk of infection. It is, therefore, important to bear this in mind when attempting to do CPR. CPR involves giving rescue breaths and providing effective chest compressions. Whilst delivering the rescue breaths and compressions is the best thing to do, you can perform just the chest compressions or hands-only compressions in the following circumstances:

NO TRAINING

If you have not received any training in CPR.

EXHAUSTION

CPR can be very exhausting. So, if you are on your own and you become exhausted while doing CPR, unfortunately, you will have to stop if you get exhausted to avoid becoming a casualty yourself. However, if you have a helper, then the best thing to do is swap with your helper every two minutes.

CASUALTY VOMITING DURING CPR

If a casualty vomits during CPR, you run the risk of choking on their vomit. You must act speedily and roll the casualty on his side away from you and allowing the vomit to completely drain out of the casualty's mouth. Check the mouth for remnants of the vomit and clear it out as much as you can, then continue CPR.

WHEN THE CHEST DOES NOT RISE WHEN YOU GIVE THE RESCUE BREATH

This may well be because of an object blocking the airway. If the chest is not rising when you deliver the rescue breath, then tilt the head and chin back and check the airway. You must check and attempt to remove the obstruction if it is visible. If you cannot see the object, do not go looking for it.

How To Minimise the Risk of Infection When Giving Rescue Breathing

Use face shields and face masks.

Face shield:

This is a plastic shield with a filter that is placed as a physical barrier between the casualty's face and your mouth. The filter is positioned around the casualty's mouth to prevent your saliva from going into his mouth and his saliva or vomit from going into your mouth.

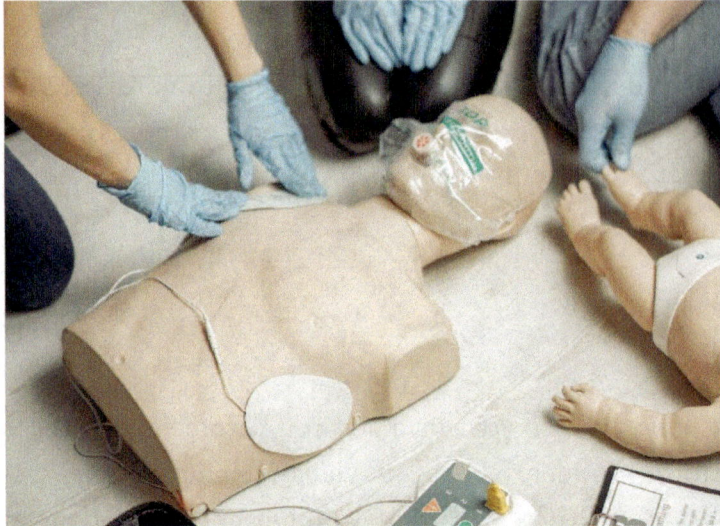

Face mask:

This is a more durable facial barrier that has a mouthpiece that is placed over the mouth of the casualty to deliver rescue breathing.

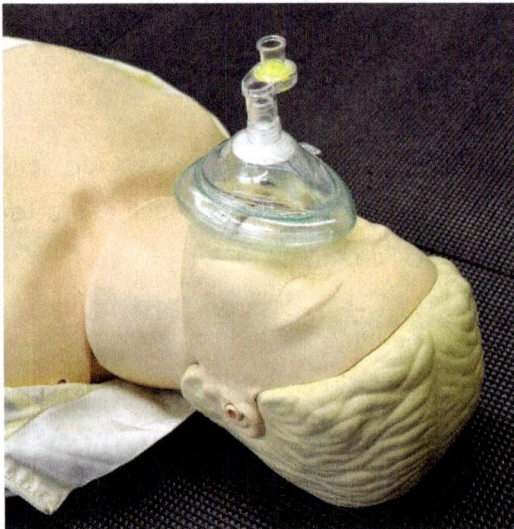

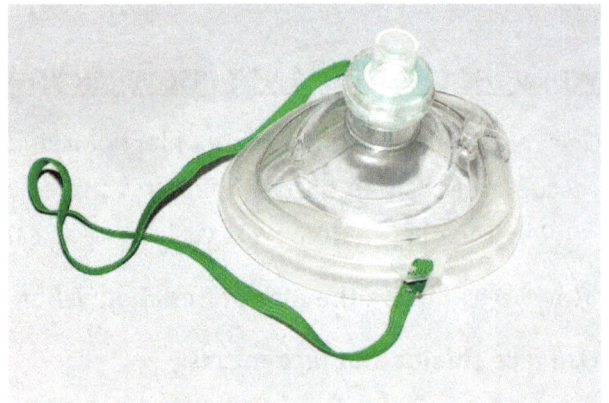

PERFORMING CPR TO A HEAVILY PREGNANT WOMAN

The effect of a heavily pregnant woman lying on her back is that the uterus will be pressing on one of the blood vessels in the abdomen, and this can lead to interruption of blood supply to the pregnant woman's heart and the result could be fatal. So, when performing CPR on a heavily pregnant woman, raise the right hip slightly so that the pregnant woman is leaning slightly to the left side. This has the effect of moving the uterus away from the blood vessel and creating an uninterrupted blood supply to her heart. A helper can assist you to raise the right hip, or if you are on your own, roll a cloth and place it under the right hip to raise it.

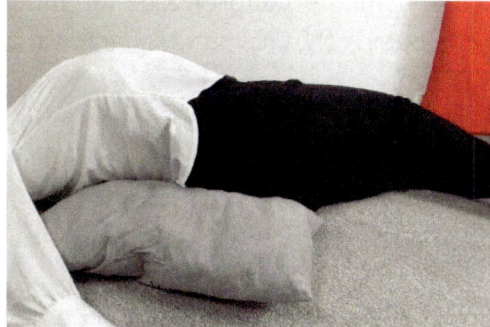

HOW TO PERFORM CPR ON A BABY

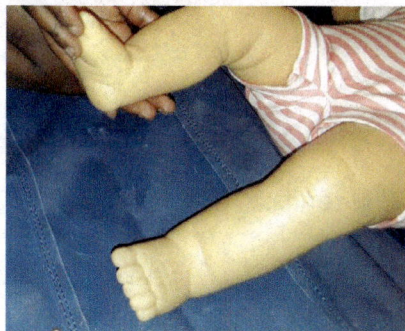

STEP 1
Lie the baby on her back on a flat surface.

STEP 2
Check if the baby is responsive by tickling their foot.

STEP 3
Open the baby's airway.

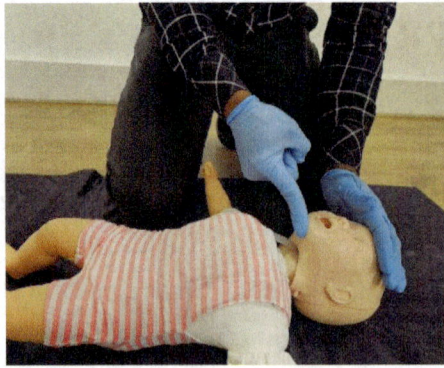

Clear the baby's airway by placing one hand on the forehead and tilting the head back gently with a finger on the free hand placed on the baby's chin. Conduct a head tilt and a chin lift.

If you can see any obstructions in the baby's mouth, remove it but do not go looking for obstructions down the throat as you may cause acute damage to the airway or push an object further down the throat.

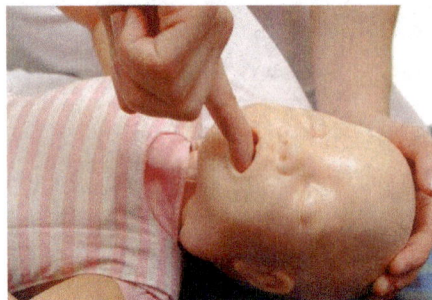

Step 4
Check if the baby is breathing for 10 seconds.

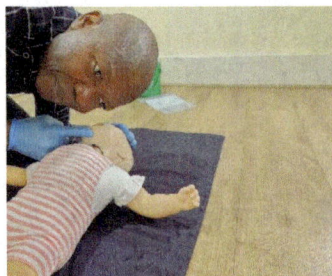

STEP 5
Give rescue breaths.

If the baby is not breathing, blow air into the baby's nose and mouth by sealing your mouth over the nose and mouth. For bigger infants where sealing your mouth over the nose and mouth is impossible, seal your mouth over the baby's nose.

Give five rescue breaths.

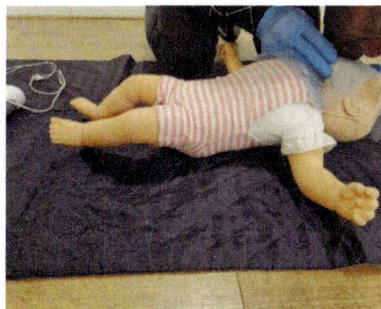

Give 30 chest compressions followed by two rescue breaths. Every chest compression you deliver should be followed by two rescue breaths.

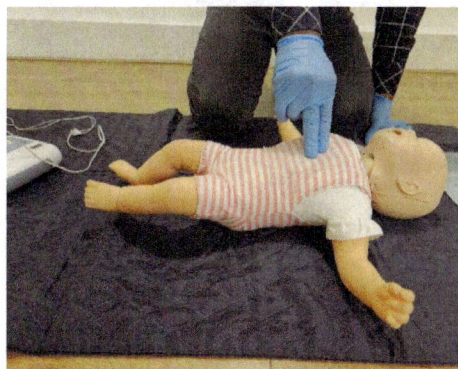

Changes you can make to the delivery of normal CPR.

- In certain circumstances, you can deliver hands-only (chest compression) CPR.

- Swap every 1-2 minutes with a helper.

- Where you deliver rescue breaths and the chest has not risen, you must recheck that the head and chin have been tilted properly. Look into the mouth to ensure there is no blockage.

- If you think rescue breaths have not been delivered effectively, have another go but do not spend more than two attempts delivering the rescue breath before conducting chest compressions.

Diverse Types of Rescue Breaths

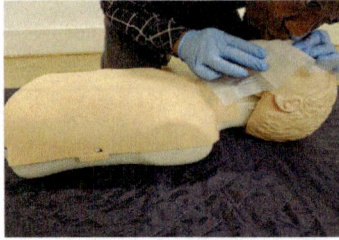

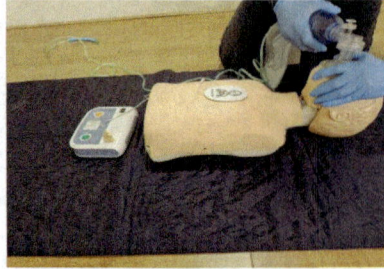

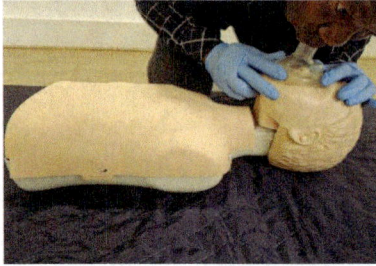

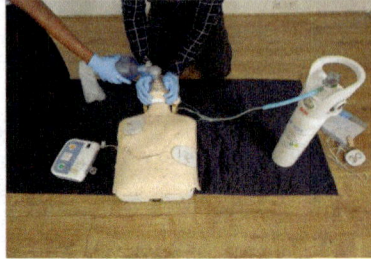

Mouth-to-mouth

This involves fully sealing your mouth over the casualty's mouth whilst, at the same time, squeezing his nose.

Circumstances when you may skip mouth-to-mouth when treating an adult:

- If the casualty's mouth is bloodied.
- If you are afraid of being infected by the casualty.
- You have not had formal training in CPR.
- You are unwilling or unable to do mouth-to-mouth.

Mouth-to-nose rescue breathing

This involves fully sealing your mouth over the casualty's nose whilst, at the same time, using your hand to cover his mouth firmly to avoid any leakage of air. When the rescue breath is delivered, allow the mouth to open so that air is released.

Circumstances when mouth-to-nose may be necessary:

- The casualty's mouth is bloodied because of an injury.
- The casualty is pulled out of water.
- The casualty is an older infant, where you are unable to seal your mouth over the infant's nose and mouth.
- You are afraid of being infected by the casualty.
- You have not had formal training in CPR.
- You are unwilling or unable to do mouth-to-mouth.

USING THE AUTOMATED EXTERNAL DEFIBRILLATOR

A heart that has stopped working is said to be in a state of cardiac arrest. This can be caused by several reasons, but the common causes are ventricular fibrillation (when the heart begins to beat like a bag of worms), and lack of oxygen to the heart. To help reset the rhythm of the heart, the casualty will benefit from the use of a defibrillator. If the casualty is not breathing, get help and send for the AED.

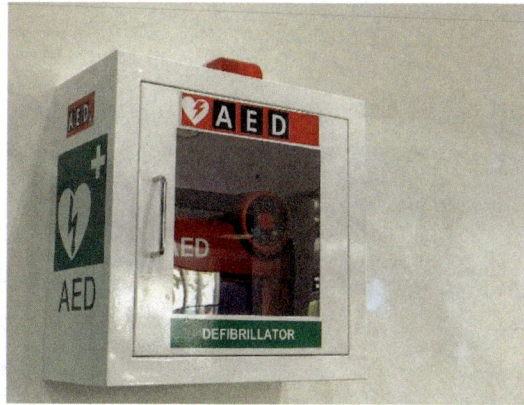

WHAT TO DO WHEN THE AED ARRIVES

Turn the machine on by pushing the on button. For most AEDs, it will be a green button.

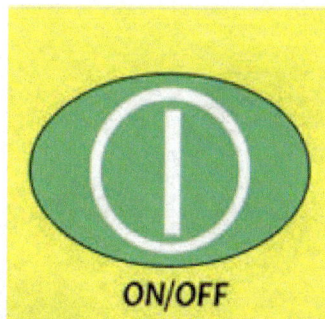

Make sure the casualty is bare-chested.

If the chest is wet, then make sure it is wiped dry. Do not spend too much time doing that.

This must be the case for all casualties, whether male or female, adult, or child. For female casualties, you will have to remove their bra—use your scissors to cut through if necessary.

Remove the electrodes or PADS from their seal and remove the backing paper to reveal the sticky part of the pads.

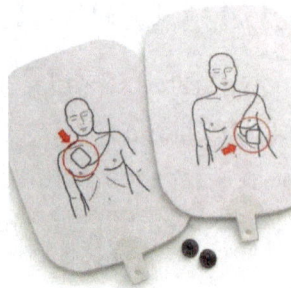

ATTACHING PADS

Place the first pad on the right part of the chest below the collarbone.

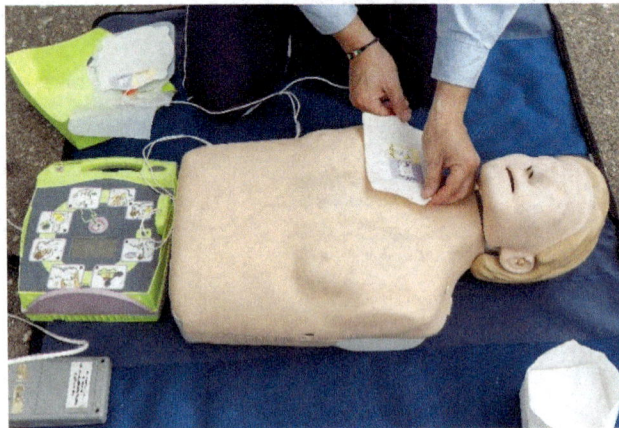

Place the second pad just below the armpit.

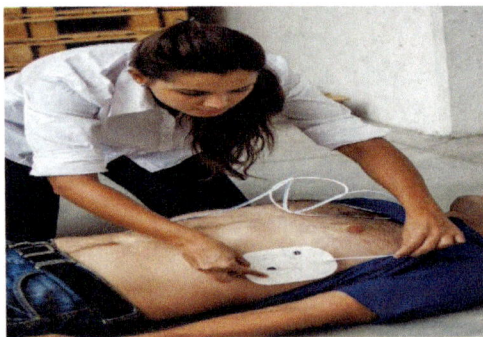

Once the pads are placed in the right positions, the machine will start analysing the heart's rhythm and follow the instructions. Semi-automatic defibrillators will usually prompt you to press a flashing orange button, which indicates the machine is ready to deliver a shock. Once you press the orange button, the machine sends an electric shock to the heart. The automatic AED will send a shock automatically. Whether automatic or semi-automatic, the machine will instruct you to stand clear before it delivers a shock. It will instruct you to administer CPR and restart analysing the heart two minutes later.

If the casualty regains consciousness, then put them in the recovery position.

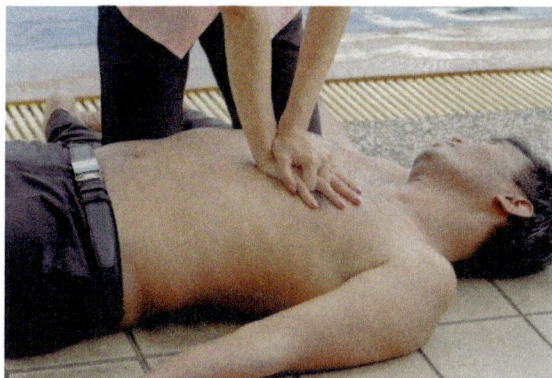

SAFETY ISSUES

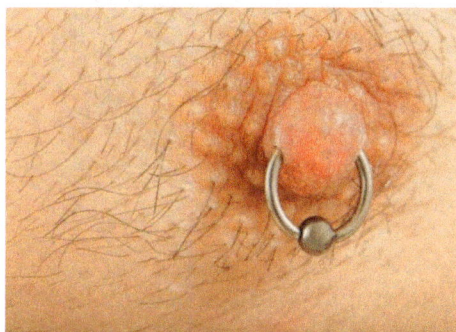

JEWELLERY

MEDICATIONS—PACEMAKER

Watch out for pacemakers. Do not place the AED pads on them.

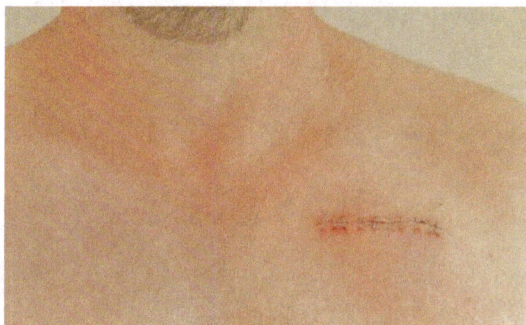

 CLOTHING

You must place the defibrillator pads on a casualty's bare chest.

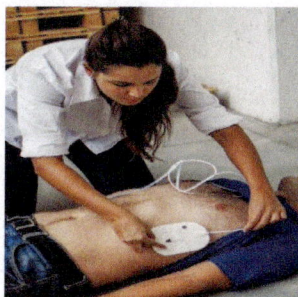

DIABETES

Diabetes is the result of damage or the ineffective functioning of the pancreas.

The pancreas is the organ that produces insulin in the body. Insulin helps cells in the body to absorb blood glucose, which is necessary for the release of metabolic energy.

Type 1 Diabetes

This is characterised by the insufficient production or lack of insulin production by the pancreas, leading to elevated

amounts of glucose in the bloodstream.

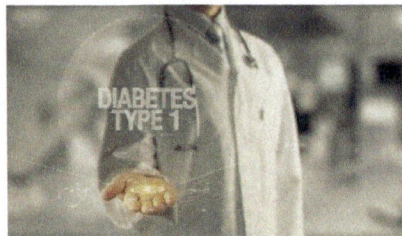

Type 2 Diabetes

This happens when the pancreas produces insulin, but the body becomes insensitive to the insulin produced by the pancreas, leading to elevated amounts of glucose in the blood.

Diabetic emergencies

Hyperglycaemia

Hyperglycaemia is a term used to describe high blood glucose levels (JRCALC).

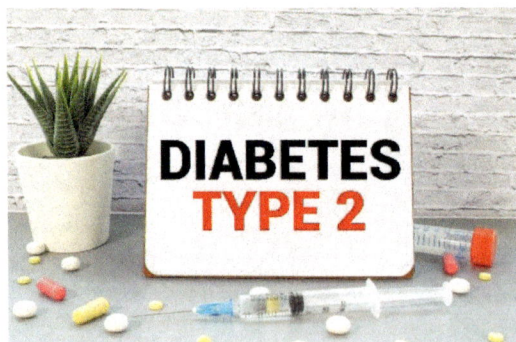

Signs and symptoms:

- Frequent urination.
- Frequent thirst.
- Tiredness.
- Those at risk of high blood sugar.
- Patients with diabetic mellitus. This is usually because of an infection.

HYPOGLYCAEMIA

- Sweating.
- Trembling/shaking.
- Palpitations.
- Headache.
- Nausea.
- Incoordination.
- Confusion.
- Speech difficulty.
- Drowsiness.
- Irrational behaviour.
- Aggressive/combative behaviour.
- Fitting.
- Unconsciousness.

Causes of Hypoglycaemia

- Administering too much insulin.
- Increased levels of exercise.
- Excessive or chronic alcohol intake.
- Inadequate carbohydrate intake.
- Increasing age.

MANAGEMENT OF HYPOGLYCAEMIA

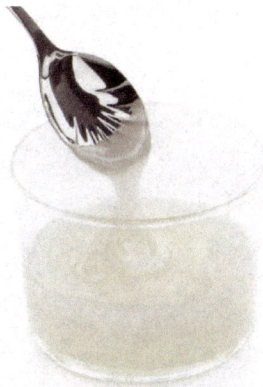

MILD TO MODERATE HYPOGLYCAEMIA

A mild to moderate patient will be conscious, oriented, and able to swallow.

ADMINISTER 15-20 GRAMS of any of the following:

- 5-7 Dextrosol tablets.

- 4-5 Glucotabs.

- 60 ml of Glucojuice.

- Or 150-200ml fruit juice e.g., orange.

- 1-2 tubes of Glucose gel.

- 3-4 teaspoons of sugar dissolved in water.

- Do not give chocolate because it is slow-acting.

- Do a glucose test after 10-15 minutes to check if blood glucose has risen to at least 4.0mmol/L and to check if the state of consciousness has improved.

- If no improvement after 30-45 minutes, then give IV glucose 19%.

- Give a starchy snack once blood glucose level hits ≥4 mmol/L. Examples of starchy snacks are two biscuits, one slice of bread/toast, and 200-300 ml glass of milk (not soya milk). Any normal meal given must contain starch. If further treatment is required, call 999 or 112.

SEIZURES

This is an abnormal electrical discharge of neurons resulting in changes in the patient's level of consciousness.

CAUSES:

- Head injury.
- Brain tumour.
- Stroke.
- Casualties who have suffered from stroke are prone to have seizures.
- Poisoning.
- Alcohol.
- Drugs.
- Heat—children are prone to this type of seizure.
- Photosensitivity.
- Flashlights trigger seizures in a sizeable number of people.

Signs and symptoms of seizures

- Preceded by an aura, which varies from patient to patient.
- Eyes rolled to the back of the head.
- Jerking movements.
- Abnormal eye movement.
- Bowel/bladder incontinence.

Management of seizures:

- Ensure the airway is clear.
- Provide supplemental oxygen.
- Make sure the patient is safe by moving them away from danger.
- Place the patient in the recovery position.
- Check the patient's vital signs.

Positional Treatment of a Seizure: Recovery Position

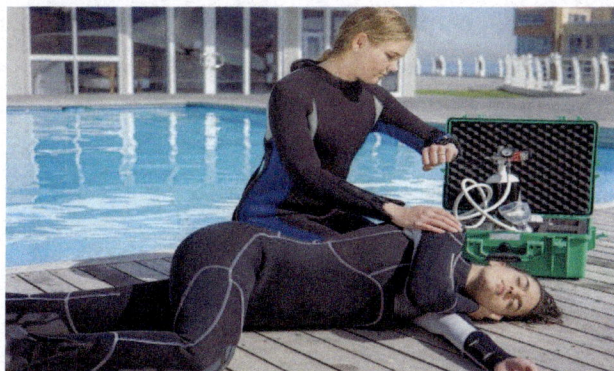

Eye Injuries

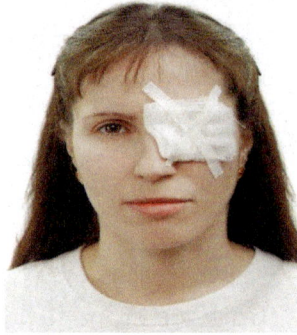

Causes of eye injuries:

Burns, chemicals, penetrating eye injury.

STROKE

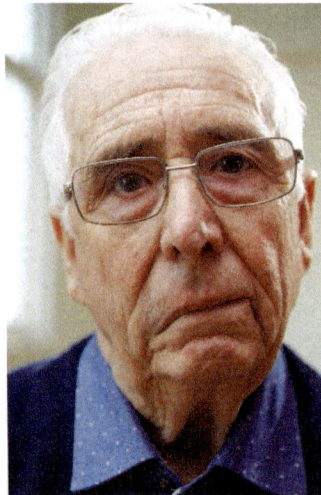

Stroke and Transient Ischaemic Attack (TIA)

A stroke can be caused by either a clot in one or more blood vessels supplying blood to the brain or a rupture in the blood vessels in the brain. Strokes are not age-specific. It can happen to anyone of any age. Time is of the essence. The speed of recovery depends on how soon the patient arrives in the hospital and receives urgent treatment.

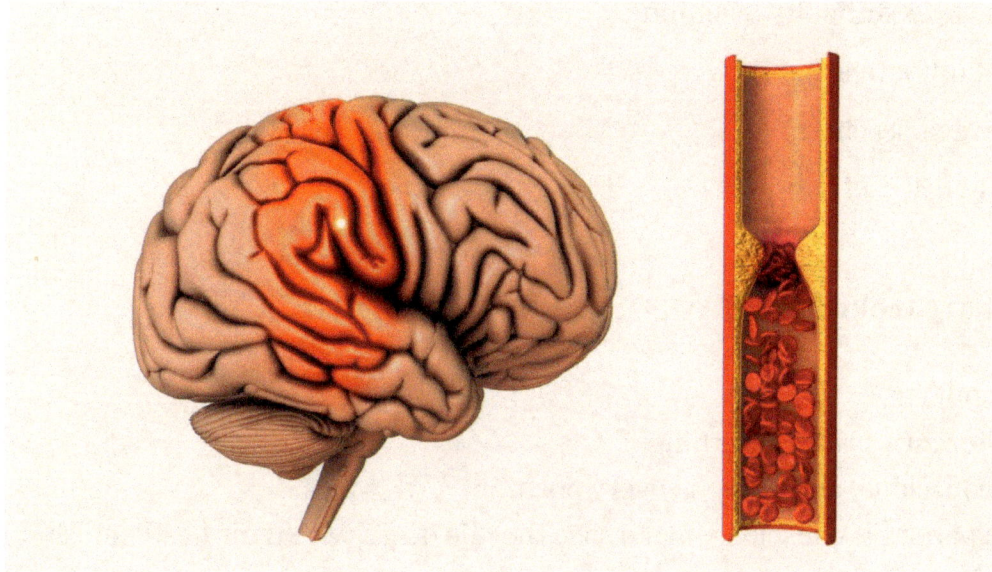

Signs and symptoms:

1. Numbness or weakness of the face, arms, or legs on either the left or right side of the body.
2. Sudden onset of seizures, syncope, sepsis, hypoglycaemia.
3. Confusion, difficulty speaking, difficulty swallowing, and difficulty understanding speech.
4. Sudden blurred vision in one or both eyes.
5. Lack of coordination and difficulty walking.
6. Severe headache.
7. Dizziness, nausea, or vomiting.
8. Sudden neck pain or neck stiffness.

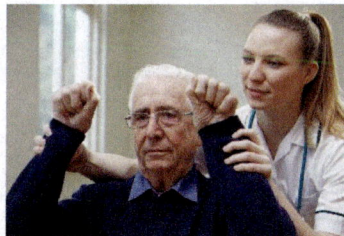

TIA

This is a temporary disruption of blood to part of the brain[1]

Always remember FAST:

---

[1] **Transient ischaemic attack (TIA) - NHS (www.nhs.uk)**

Face: Droopy face, difficulty in smiling.

Arm: Cannot lift both arms.

Speech: Slurred speech.

Time: Time to call 999/112.

Treatment of Stroke and TIA:

- Call 999/112.
- Monitor airway and breathing.
- If unconscious, place in a recovery position.
- If the patient is conscious, make sure they lie down with their head and shoulders raised.
- Monitor vital signs—breathing, pulse, and level of response while waiting for help.
- Nil by mouth. Do not give drinks or food to the patient as it may be difficult for the patient to swallow.

FIRST AID KIT

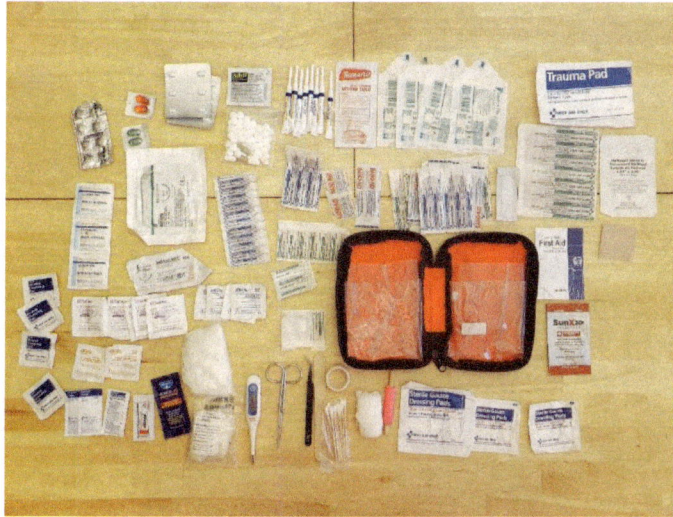

FIRST AID KIT RESOURCE SHEET

Have you ever tried to get a plaster from a first aid kit only to discover there is none? If only someone had completed this first aid resource sheet, then a first aider responsible for checking the first aid kit would have replenished it to avoid the shortage.

FIRST AID KIT RESOURCE SHEET

DAY   DATE:

Item	Time	No. in box	Number Taken	Items Left	Replaced On	Items Left	First Aider
Guidance Leaflet							
Wash-Proof Plasters							
Eye Pads							

Triangular Bandage	
Safety Pins	
Dressings 12×12cm	
Dressings 18×18cm	
Moist Wipes	
Disposable Gloves	
Scissors (Tuff Cuts)	

ISBN   978-1-7385061-4-9

9 781738 506149 >

Printed in Dunstable, United Kingdom